# The Lung: Molecular Basis of Disease

. . . . . . . . . . . . . . . . . . . . . .

# The Lung: Molecular Basis of Disease

· · · · · · · · · · · · · · · · · · · · ·

## JEROME S. BRODY, MD

Professor of Medicine
Director, Pulmonary Center
Vice-Chairman of Medicine Research
Boston University School of Medicine
Boston, Massachusetts

## W.B. Saunders Company

*A Division of Harcourt Brace & Company*

Philadelphia London Toronto Montreal Sydney Tokyo

**W.B. SAUNDERS COMPANY**
*A Division of Harcourt Brace & Company*

The Curtis Center
Independence Square West
Philadelphia, Pennsylvania 19106

WF
600
B865m
1998

**Library of Congress Cataloging-in-Publication Data**

The Lung: Molecular Basis of Disease / Jerome S. Brody.—1st ed.

p.    cm.

Includes bibliographical references.

ISBN 0-7216-6814-3

1. Respiratory organs—Diseases—Molecular aspects.    2. Amyotrophic
   lateral sclerosis—Molecular aspects.    I. Title.    [DNLM: 1. Lung
   Diseases—genetics.    2. Amyotrophic Lateral Sclerosis—genetics.
   3. Molecular Biology.    4. Gene Therapy.    WF 600 B865m 1998]

RC711.B76 1998      617.5′407—dc21

DNLM/DLC                                                        97-27841

THE LUNG: MOLECULAR BASIS OF DISEASE

ISBN 0-7216-6814-3

Printed in the United States of America.

Last digit is the print number:    9    8    7    6    5    4    3    2    1

This book is dedicated to my wife,

Annie, and to my children,

Lisa, Karen, Marion, Leah, and David.

Annie is both the reason it took so

long to write this book and the

reason I was able to finish it. She

provided emotional support and

much-needed nagging

in the right amounts at the right time.

# Preface

· · · · · · · · · · · · · · · · · · · · · · ·

Molecular biology (the study of gene structure and function) has undergone an amazing evolution over the past 40 years, from the discovery of the three-dimensional structure of DNA in the 1950s to the development of human gene therapy and genetically engineered drugs in the 1990s. This evolution has taken place in three major phases: (1) discovery of basic concepts of DNA, RNA, and genetic code in the 1950s; (2) discovery of a number of tools that allowed practical manipulation of DNA and RNA in the 1970s; and (3) publication of texts and "cookbooks" and availability of "do it yourself" kits in the 1980s and 1990s, which popularized molecular biology so that it could be applied to clinical medicine. Thus, molecular biology and its powerful tools, once the exclusive domain of physical chemists, biochemists, and geneticists, have now entered the world of the clinician, and the basic methods used by molecular biologists are responsible for an increasing number of articles that now appear in clinical journals. Recognizing the importance of this "new science" in clinical medicine, several journals have begun to present reviews of basic concepts for clinicians.

This is one of the most exciting times in medical science, with new basic discoveries happening weekly. Progress now occurs so rapidly that the time from basic discovery to clinical application can be measured in months, yet, paradoxically, it seems to me that most clinicians are increasingly distanced from the science being applied to their patients and from the discoveries that almost daily appear in lay journals and newspapers. This trend of distance from the "new science" has accelerated with the pressures on institutions responsible for training physicians to turn out more primary care givers and fewer academic physicians whose focus is on the basic biology of disease. Academic medical centers seem to be moving toward a bimodal distribution of faculty and trainees—primary health care deliverers and basic scientists —with the practical and psychological distance between them widening just when discoveries in the laboratory are moving closer to potential clinical application.

At the present time, pulmonary medicine is reminiscent of the mid-1950s when Julius Comroe and his colleagues wrote their highly influential primer, *The Lung: Clinical Physiology and Pulmonary Function Tests*. Comroe's reason for writing *The Lung* was much the same as mine for writing this book. To paraphrase his preface, with molecular biology being substituted for physiology: "Pulmonary scientists who use physiological [*molecular biologic*] techniques understand physiology [*molecular biology*] reasonably well. Many pulmonary doctors and trainees do not. One reason is that most pulmonary scientists, in their original and review articles, write for other scientists and not for doctors and medical students. This is not a book for pulmonary scientists; it is written for doctors and students. Its purpose is to explain in simple words and diagrams those aspects of physiology [*molecular biology*] that are important to clinical medicine, particularly pulmonary medicine." This book is not meant to compete with a number of excellent texts that teach cell and molecular biology. Rather it is meant to provide sufficient background to enable physicians and students to understand how molecular biology is now impacting on pulmonary practice and to be able to understand the coming advances in pulmonary medicine that will require familiarity with concepts of molecular biology. My goal is not to teach about disease using the principles of molecular biology, but to use pulmonary diseases to teach the basics of molecular biology. I plan both to present molecular biology concepts and to explain how molecular biology data are obtained.

Molecular biology can be intimidating, as was pulmonary physiology a generation or two ago (and still is to many). The language is mystifying and often whimsical, and the concepts are so foreign as to discourage most physicians, especially those who grew up learning the cutting edge physiology of the 1950s and 1960s, from even reading the abstracts of articles based on molecular biology. That cutting edge of 1950 to 1960 science, demystified in *The Lung*, became the bedside medicine of the present era, just as molecular biology and cutting-edge science of the present decade will become the bedside medicine of the next generation. When I needed to check whether I understood some pulmonary physiology concept such as physiologic dead space in order to read a clinical article, I always went back to *The Lung* for a clear explanation. I hope that *The Lung: Molecular Basis of Disease* will be the same for pulmonary physicians struggling to understand what a knockout is or how one screens a library.

The format of this book is somewhat similar to that of *The Lung*. Following a chapter introducing basic concepts of molecular biology, a series of chapters illustrate these principles and introduce additional concepts as they have been applied to specific pulmonary diseases. The first chapter, called The Basics, covers the basic concepts of what DNA is and how it is organized to govern the making of proteins. The polymerase chain reaction is explained by discussing its application to the diagnosis of tuberculosis. Concepts such as cloning DNA and screening libraries are illustrated in discussions of virulence and drug resistance in the chapter on tuberculosis. The chapter on amyotrophic lateral sclerosis provides an opportunity to discuss the structure of chromosomes and concepts of how to find a gene by linkage analysis. It also presents an opportunity to explain transgenic mice and site-directed mutagenesis. The etiology of pulmonary alveolar proteinosis has been clarified using methods based on homologous recombination and gene targeting that produced a knockout of a gene that appears to be involved in surfactant recycling. Cystic fibrosis is used to discuss deduction of protein structure from gene sequence. It is also used as a clinical model for illustrating principles having to do with genetic screening and, of course, is used to discuss gene therapy, since it has been the disease that has generated the most vigorous application of molecular biologic tools in all of clinical medicine. Lung cancer provides an opportunity to discuss DNA replication, oncogenes and anti-oncogenes, and DNA mutations. The chapter on developmental biology of the lung illustrates concepts of cell-specific gene regulation, transcription factors, and transgenic animals. The book ends with a discussion of the human genome. Each chapter begins with a list of basic concepts to be discussed and ends with a limited number of selected references. No attempt has been made to present a comprehensive analysis of the molecular basis of each disease. Rather, each chapter begins with a brief summary of the "state of the art." The Appendix contains a glossary of terms with definitions.

The rapid pace at which tools of molecular biology have been applied to clinical medicine guarantees that new concepts, new methods, and new and exciting discoveries relating to pulmonary medicine will likely occur while this book is in press. However, most of the principles illustrated in this book will not change dramatically. As with *The Lung* and physiology, I hope this book can be used for some time as an introduction to molecular biology, a discipline that will undoubtedly become the foundation on which clinical pulmonary medicine of the next generation will be based.

JEROME S. BRODY, MD

# Acknowledgments

. . . . . . . . . . . . . . . . . . . . . . . .

I wish to thank my former *Red Journal* co-editor Bob Senior for his critical reading of the first draft of this book and for his enthusiastic support when I needed it the most. I also thank Buddy Hammerman for his critical review and Mary Williams and the members of the Boston University Pulmonary Center for their suggestions, for the many discussions we had about the content of this book, and for helping to create the intellectual atmosphere that made it easy to write about molecular biology and the lung.

# Contents

· · · · · · · · · · · · · · · · · · · · ·

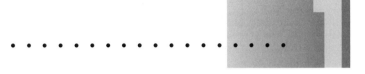

# The Basics

DNA • RNA • mRNA • nucleic acids • genetic
code • transcription • translation • gene •
genome • probes • hybridization • Southern,
Northern, Western blots

## The Central Dogma

All the information that is necessary for the formation of cells and tissues, for cell proliferation and differentiation, and for synthesis and processing of the proteins, lipids, and sugars that we are made of is stored in DNA. This genetic information is copied or transcribed into RNA, which then confers or translates the information into proteins whose synthesis is directed by RNA (Fig. 1–1). DNA does not take part directly in protein synthesis because it is in chromosomes in the nucleus, and protein synthesis occurs in the cytoplasm. Therefore, an intermediate is required that faithfully transfers the genetic information of DNA to the site of protein synthesis. A form of RNA, called messenger RNA (mRNA), is the vehicle for carrying the information or message stored in DNA. Pre-mRNA is synthesized as an exact complementary copy of DNA (see later for discussion of complementarity); it is processed to eliminate information that exists in DNA but is not necessary for protein synthesis. The fully processed RNA (mRNA) is transported to the cytoplasm, where it associates with two other forms of RNA, ribosomal RNA (rRNA) and transfer RNA (tRNA), in order to translate the DNA message into a newly synthesized protein. This protein then undergoes biochemical processing to

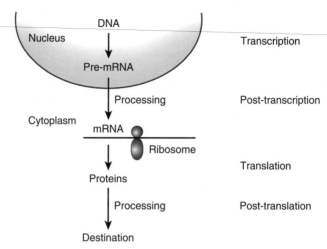

FIGURE 1–1. **The Central Dogma: DNA to RNA to Protein.** DNA is transcribed into a nuclear form of RNA, which is then post-transcriptionally processed by removal of information that is not required for protein synthesis. The product, mRNA, is transported to the cytoplasm, where it associates with ribosomes and translates the information encoded in its nucleic acids into proteins, which are then post-translationally processed to produce the final products.

assume its final structure and be sent to the site at which it performs its functions.

The making of RNA is called transcription because the genetic information encoded in DNA is transcribed to mRNA. Everything that happens after DNA is transcribed is post-transcriptional. The making of protein from mRNA is called translation—translation of the genetic code. The modifications that occur in protein (e.g., glycosylation) are post-translational modifications.

The proteins synthesized include enzymes that regulate many biologic processes, including the synthesis of lipids and carbohydrates that are not directly programmed by the genetic information in DNA. Other proteins that are synthesized are processed and secreted, are used in the cytoplasm, or return to the nucleus to participate in and, in some cases, regulate DNA-related functions.

DNA consists of four bases (two purines and two pyrimidines) that, through variation in their appearance on the DNA chain, create combinations that in humans form some 50,000 to 100,000 genes packed tightly into the nucleus of all of the cells on 23 chromosomes (Fig. 1–2). A *gene* is that segment of DNA that is sufficient to *encode* (provide the information for making) a specific protein. The four bases, in a triplet sequence, provide a genetic code that, through RNA, designates 1 of 20 amino acids. Each triplet specifies a particular amino acid (although more than one triplet can encode a given amino acid), and these amino acids, in turn, are organized to form the large number of proteins that determine how our bodies function. The

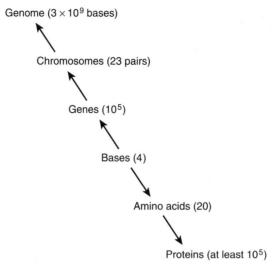

Genome ($3 \times 10^9$ bases)

Chromosomes (23 pairs)

Genes ($10^5$)

Bases (4)

Amino acids (20)

Proteins (at least $10^5$)

FIGURE 1–2. **The Central Dogma: Just Four Bases Make $10^5$ Genes.** The four nucleotides (thymine, cytosine, guanine, and adenine) combine to code for the 50,000 to 100,000 genes that make up the human genome. These genes are arranged on the 23 pairs of chromosomes to make up the human genome of more than 1 billion base pairs.

protein-coding portion of DNA occupies only a small portion of the total genome, which consists of $3 \times 10^9$ base pairs. Much of the information in the genome contains important "noncoding" information that provides directions such as when or where a gene is to be transcribed. In addition, there is a considerable amount of DNA in the human genome (perhaps the majority of DNA) whose function has yet to be defined, and this DNA is currently called "junk." This junk has likely accumulated during evolution and may provide information about the evolutionary process because simpler organisms have much less of it than humans do.

A recent review in *Scientific American* provides an analogy that helps put the genome in perspective. Every cell has within it the entire "manual" of all the information needed to make a human being. However, each cell uses only a small part of the manual to carry out its specific functions. The manual can be thought of as the human genome. It is written in a language, or more accurately a code, that uses only four letters, A, C, G, and T, which stand for the nucleotides adenine, cytosine, guanine, and thymine. During each cell division, the entire manual is reproduced so that each daughter cell has a copy. This is no small task because the complete manual consists of 3 billion pairs of letters or nucleotides. If these letters were printed on a standard-sized page that can carry 3000 letters, the manual would occupy 1000 volumes, each volume consisting of 1000 pages, and all of this fits within the nucleus of every human cell.

## DNA Structure

DNA consists of two strands of nucleotides, which are nitrogen ring structures (or bases) connected to deoxyribose sugars. These strands coil around one another in a clockwise direction to form a helix; since there are two strands, DNA exists as the now famous *double helix* (Fig. 1–3). The sugars in each chain are connected by phosphodiester bonds that form links between the 5′ carbon on one sugar and the 3′ carbon on the next, producing the regularly structured backbone of DNA. This 5′ to 3′ connection gives DNA an orientation that guides the synthesis of DNA and that of RNA, which always proceeds from the 5′ beginning of the gene to the 3′ end of the gene. The DNA chains are linked to one another by hydrogen bonds connecting bases that lie on the inside of the helix facing one another (Fig. 1–4). The two chains coil around one another in a clockwise fashion; one strand runs in a 5′ to 3′ direction (the anitisense strand that is copied into RNA), and the other runs in a 3′ to 5′ direction (the sense strand).

In contrast to the regular repeating chain of deoxyribose sugars, the sequence of the four bases that connect the DNA chains is greatly varied. Indeed it is the variation in the combinations of these bases that is responsible for the genetic code of DNA. The bases are either purines that have two rings or pyrimidines that have a single ring. It is remarkable that there are only four bases that carry all the genetic information of DNA—two purines, A and G (adenine and guanine), and two pyrimidines, C and T (cytosine and thymine). One purine always pairs with a pyrimidine base on the opposite chain in a predictable fashion; G (guanine) pairs only with C (cytosine), whereas A (adenine) pairs only with T (thymidine) (see Figs. 1–3 and 1–4). This obligatory pairing of bases, determined by their hydrogen bonding, ensures that if one strand of DNA has a G base, the complementary strand will connect via a C base. If one set of bases is known, the bases on the complementary strand can be predicted. This specific pairing of bases, called complementarity, is fundamental to understanding how DNA strands form and are replicated and how DNA transfers its information to RNA. It guarantees the faithful reproduction of DNA sequences when DNA is copied or repaired and the accurate transmission of the genetic code when DNA is being transcribed into RNA. Complementarity of DNA bases is also fundamental to techniques such as Northern and Southern blots, which measure RNA and DNA; the polymerase chain reaction; screening DNA libraries; and most of the other molecular techniques to be discussed later. If one set of bases is known, one can construct a complementary set of bases that will selectively bind to the first set. If the constructed set of bases has radioactivity incorporated into it, its complementary strand will be labeled with radioactivity.

The DNA strands also form a template on which DNA is replicated during cell division. During this process, the DNA strands separate and new complementary strands are formed. The new strands then combine to form new DNA helices (see Chapter 7).

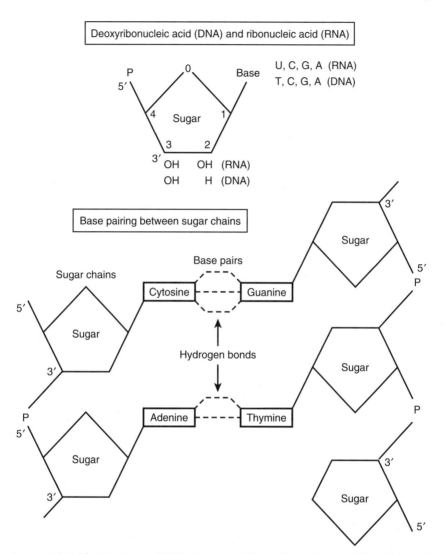

FIGURE 1–3. **The Structure of DNA: Sugars and Bases.** Deoxyribose and ribonucleic acids are pentose sugars with phosphates in the 5′ position and one of four different bases. RNA differs from DNA in that uridine is substituted for thymidine. DNA consists of pentose sugars linked together in strands via phosphates. The two pentose strands are linked by hydrogen bonds that form between bases that always pair in a C to G and A to T fashion. Guanine and adenine are purines and cytosine and thymine are pyrimidines.

## How DNA Is Organized

DNA is not continuously transcribed into RNA. Many proteins are required only when cells are called on to perform specific functions, for example, cell division, production of matrix proteins, synthesis of cytokines, and so on. Thus

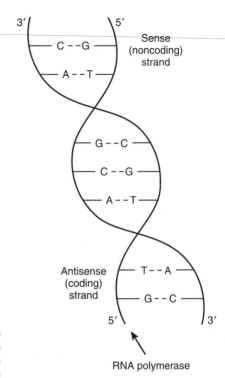

FIGURE 1–4. **The DNA Double Helix.** The two DNA strands intertwine to form a double helix, with one strand in a 5′ to 3′ orientation (the antisense, coding strand) and the other in a 3′ to 5′ orientation (the sense, noncoding strand). RNA polymerase catalyzes the reading of the antisense strand, producing an exact copy of the sense strand.

DNA must contain information that regulates its state of transcription. These components provide binding sites for cellular proteins (*trans*-acting [across] factors) that interact with specific areas of the DNA (*cis*-acting [on this side] elements), forming complexes that then initiate transcription. The sites that initiate transcription and the proteins that bind to these sites tend to be shared by many genes. These regions, which are generally close to the site at which transcription is initiated, are called promoters. A complex of transcription factors assemble here, providing a place where RNA polymerase can bind and initiate transcription (Fig. 1–5).

There are also binding sites that are unique to specific DNA molecules. These sites, to which proteins also bind, can be some distance from the initiation site, either 5′ or 3′ to the initiation site. They can be *enhancers* that upregulate transcription or *silencers* that downregulate transcription. More than one protein is usually involved in activating an enhancer or silencer. This system of general and cell-specific transcription factors, which can act in either a positive or a negative fashion, provides a mechanism for regulating

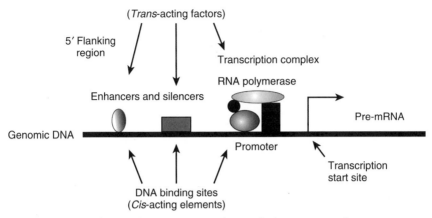

FIGURE 1–5. **Regulation of Transcription: The 5′ Flanking Region of Genomic DNA.** The region of DNA 5′ to the transcription start site contains regulatory elements (*cis*-acting elements) that serve as binding sites for *trans*-acting transcription factors that regulate transcription of the DNA. A promoter region, which usually lies 50 to 150 base pairs upstream of the start site, is a focus for assembly of the proteins that make up the basal transcription complex. RNA polymerase, which is the enzyme that copies the antisense DNA strand, is part of this complex. Other *trans*-acting proteins serve to enhance or silence the activity of the basal transcription complex.

cell-specific gene expression and protein synthesis. This process is discussed in more detail in Chapter 8.

The gene regulatory information in DNA is eliminated in producing mRNA because it is irrelevant to translation, which is the main job of mRNA. DNA also contains information in introns that are downstream, or 3′, to the transcription start site, and this information is copied or transcribed into the pre-mRNA that is produced initially but is not present in the fully processed mRNA that enters the cytoplasm. Introns contain gene regulatory information and likely serve other functions that are not well understood and are not preserved in mRNA. *Exons* are the code-containing regions of DNA that are preserved in mRNA and serve to dictate protein synthesis. However, not all exons are actually translated. Exons that appear before or after the actual coding region (see further on) are in the 5′ *or 3′ untranslated region* and serve to regulate translation (Fig. 1–6).

## Transcription of DNA Information to RNA and RNA Structure

DNA is a stable molecule. When DNA is injured as a result of an environmental insult, it is repaired. When cells divide during growth or repair of tissue damage, DNA is replicated. At other times, however, there is no DNA synthesis. In contrast, mRNA is not stable; it is degraded once made. There-

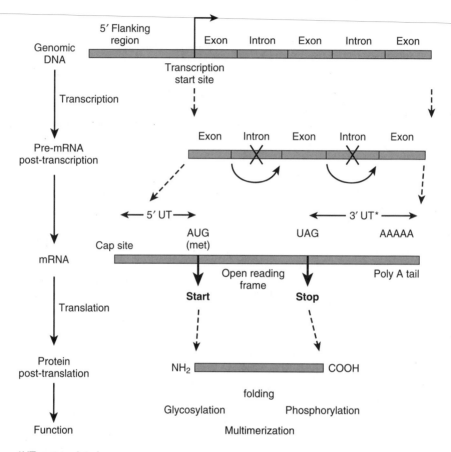

*UT=untranslated

FIGURE 1–6. **Another View of DNA, RNA, and Protein Processing and Structure.** Genomic DNA has a 5′ flanking region, a transcription start site that determines where RNA polymerase begins the transcription process, and a set of introns and exons that are downstream from the start site. Exons remain in the final processed mRNA. Introns that may contain transcriptional regulatory information are eliminated in the post-transcriptional processing of pre-mRNA. mRNA has both a 5′ and a 3′ untranslated region flanking the mRNA coding region or open reading frame. The first ribonucleotide at the 5′ end is modified to form a cap that protects the 5′ end from degradation. The 3′ end usually has a string of AAAs that form the so-called poly A tail, which among other things serves to stabilize mRNA. The open reading frame, which is the start site for translation of the mRNA into protein, always begins with the three-letter code for methionine and ends with a three-letter code (the stop code) that does not signal for an amino acid. Once mRNA is translated into a protein with an amino and a carboxyl terminus, it undergoes post-translational modification to assume its final shape and function. This function may require homodimerization, heterodimerization or multimerization, that is, interaction with itself or other proteins in complexes of various sizes. Glycosylation or phosphorylation of amino acids may also occur. It is these latter post-translational modifications that affect the final function of the protein.

fore, new RNA is required every time a protein is synthesized. Thus, when a protein is needed, transcription takes place; in the presence of continued protein synthesis, RNA must be transcribed continuously.

RNA exists as a single strand that is identical to the sense strand of DNA, except that its backbone sugar is ribose rather than deoxyribose and one of its bases, uracil, substitutes for thymine in DNA. There is no RNA helix, but RNA can assume a secondary structure that serves to influence its function. There are three types of fully processed RNA, all of which function in the cytoplasm rather than the nucleus. The RNA that carries the genetic message of DNA that is translated into proteins, mRNA, actually accounts for less than 5% of total RNA. The other two RNA types, rRNA and tRNA, are also involved in the formation of proteins (see later discussion of translation) and account for 80% and 15% of total RNA, respectively.

RNA formation requires the initiation of DNA transcription and the presence of the enzyme *RNA polymerase*. This enzyme catalyzes the copying of the DNA template into RNA. This occurs in a 5' to 3' direction; thus RNA polymerase reads the antisense strand of DNA and reproduces the sense strand (see Fig. 1–4). The RNA chain contains bases that are complementary to the DNA bases, that is, the base sequence GTACG on DNA is copied as CAUGC on RNA (remember U in RNA substitutes for T in DNA). In all cases the RNA that is first made must be extensively modified before it is transferred to the cytoplasm to perform its functions.

Three RNA polymerase enzymes are involved in the synthesis of the three types of RNA involved in making proteins. In the presence of transcription factors (see previous discussion) and RNA polymerase, which opens the DNA for copying, RNA synthesis proceeds in a 5' to 3' direction as noted earlier. The transcription complex traverses the entire gene, often tens or hundreds of thousands of base pairs. At the end of the DNA, a termination site is recognized and the complex dissociates from the DNA template. The product of RNA polymerase I is rRNA, which provides the scaffold on which mRNA directs assembly of proteins. RNA polymerase III catalyzes the transcription of tRNA, which carries specific amino acids to the ribosome on which the peptide chain of proteins is assembled.

Polymerase II regulates transcription of the RNA that carries the genetic message of DNA to the cytoplasm for translation into protein. This RNA is called pre-mRNA or, more accurately, heterogeneous nuclear RNA (hnRNA) when it is in the nucleus and mRNA after it is modified and transported to the cytoplasm. RNA, when first transcribed, is an accurate and faithful copy of DNA minus the 5' flanking region of DNA that regulates RNA transcription (see Fig. 1–6). However, as noted earlier, this pre-mRNA undergoes considerable post-transcriptional processing before it is transported to the cytoplasm as the mature mRNA that directs translation. Figure 1–7 shows that the mRNA encoding the cystic fibrosis transport regulator (CFTR), a 167,000-kd protein, is 6500 base pairs (6.5 kilobases [kb]), containing much more information than is necessary to account for the actual protein. The

## *CFTR* FROM GENE TO PROTEIN

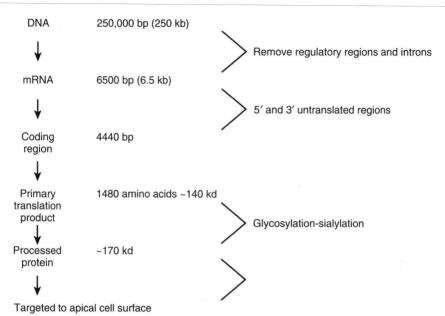

DNA — 250,000 bp (250 kb)

↓ Remove regulatory regions and introns

mRNA — 6500 bp (6.5 kb)

↓ 5′ and 3′ untranslated regions

Coding region — 4440 bp

↓

Primary translation product — 1480 amino acids ~140 kd

↓ Glycosylation-sialylation

Processed protein — ~170 kd

↓

Targeted to apical cell surface

FIGURE 1–7. **Processing, from Gene to Protein: the Example of *CFTR*.** The figure shows the change in size of DNA and RNA as *CFTR* is processed. Genomic DNA contains 244 base pairs of regulatory information and "junk" whose function is not known. The mRNA open reading frame codes for a primary translation product of 1480 amino acids, which is then post-translationally modified to form a 170-kd protein that is normally targeted to the apical cell surface of epithelial cells. The last step in the process is altered in the most common form of *CFTR* mutation (see Chapter 6).

mRNA is copied from a DNA molecule that is 250,000 base pairs (250 kb), 40 times the size of the 6.5-kb mRNA. Thus a considerable amount of post-transcriptional processing of hnRNA occurs before it is ready to be transported as mRNA from the nucleus to the cytoplasm. The major steps in the processing of pre-mRNA include splicing out the noncoding introns and joining the exons (some 27 exons for CFTR), capping the 5′ end of the spliced mRNA, and adding a run of AAAA nucleotides at the 3′ end of RNA forming the poly A tail of mRNA. The 5′ capping modification of RNA protects the forming RNA from degradation and provides a site that will be important in the initiation of protein synthesis. The addition of a poly A tail to the 3′ end affects a number of events, including mRNA transport to the cytoplasm, mRNA stability, and recognition of rRNA in the cytoplasm. Splicing out introns occurs within nuclear spliceosomes. This is a complex process discussed further in Chapter 6.

The fully processed mRNA (see Fig. 1–6) contains a "cap site" at its 5′ end and a poly A tail added to the 3′ end of the mRNA. The processed mRNA also contains a 5′ upstream region and a 3′ downstream region that do not translate into protein and are thus called 5′ and 3′ untranslated regions. The functions of these regions are not completely clear, but they appear to regulate the effectiveness of mRNA translation and its stability. Downstream of the 5′ untranslated region, mRNA contains a triplet nucleotide code, or *codon*, which signals the initiation of translation; farther downstream is a codon that signals termination of translation. The region of mRNA between the initiation and termination signals is the coding region or open reading frame, which actually contains the code for the protein to be made. The mature mRNA is rapidly transported to the cytoplasm through pores in the nuclear membrane and appears immediately to associate with proteins that link it to the ribosome. Ribosome collections in the cytoplasm are the site of most protein synthesis, but those proteins that are to be secreted or transported to the cell membrane move, after the addition of a signal peptide, to the endoplasmic reticulum (ER), where synthesis is completed.

## Translation of the Message: Making a Protein

The mRNA bases are the key to a code that specifies which amino acids are to be incorporated into the protein being made and in what sequence the amino acids are to appear. The combination of three of the four bases (A,T,U, and C) provides a three-letter code, or codon, which specifies 1 of the 20 amino acids (Fig. 1–8). There are 64 possible combinations of the four bases for the 20 amino acids. Thus the coding system is redundant (or *degenerate*) in that some amino acids can be coded for by more than one combination of bases. The codon AUG specifies methionine, which is the clue to start translation. Usually a special sequence of bases precedes the AUG start codon, thus additionally fixing the site at which protein synthesis begins. The codons UAA, UGA, and UAG do not specify any amino acid and thus act as a signal for the termination of translation and the end of the protein being made (Fig. 1–9; see also Fig. 1–8).

Each of the RNA types described previously participates in the translation process. *mRNA* provides the codon-based genetic code that determines the sequence of amino acids in the protein to be made (Fig. 1–10). *rRNA* forms a complex, the ribosome, which is the structure in which the components of the protein synthetic process assemble. The ribosome moves along the mRNA template, providing a positioning mechanism for *tRNA* to bring the appropriate amino acid to the lengthening chain that forms the growing (nascent) peptide.

An initiation factor binds the methionine tRNA, and this complex serves to bring other initiation factors to mRNA using the cap site and to the small ribosomal subunit. The ribosome is guided to the initiation site by the short nucleotide sequence that precedes the AUG start codon. The large subunit joins this complex and translation begins.

mRNA coding sequences for amino acids

| Position 1 | Position 2 | | | | Position 3 |
|---|---|---|---|---|---|
| | U | C | A | G | |
| U | phe | ser | tyr | cys | U |
| | phe | ser | try | cys | C |
| | leu | ser | stop | stop | A |
| | leu | ser | stop | trp | G |
| C | leu | pro | his | arg | U |
| | leu | pro | his | arg | C |
| | leu | pro | gln | arg | A |
| | leu | pro | gln | arg | G |
| A | ile | thr | asn | ser | U |
| | ile | thr | asn | ser | C |
| | ile | thr | lys | arg | A |
| | met | thr | lys | arg | G |
| G | val | ala | asp | gly | U |
| | val | ala | asp | gly | C |
| | val | ala | glu | gly | A |
| | val | ala | glu | gly | G |

Code for: Tryptophan: UGG
Methionine: AUG
Phenylalanine: UU*U* or UU*C*
Glutamine: GA*A* or GA*G*
Leucine: CU*U* or CU*C* or CU*A* or CU*G*
Arginine: CG*U* or CG*C* or CG*A* or CG*G* or *AG*A or *AG*G

FIGURE 1–8. **The Genetic Code: Which Nucleotides for Which Amino Acids?** The figure illustrates the three-letter codons for the 20 amino acids. There is only one code for methionine, the start codon for translation of mRNA. Several codons do not call for an amino acid (UAA, UAG, and UGA) and therefore signify an end to translation. Some amino acids are highly degenerate, that is, they can be signified by a number of different codons. In most of these instances, the third letter of the code is the one that can change without affecting the amino acid produced (see arginine *[arg]*).

The first amino acid, methionine, forms the amino terminal of the nascent peptide and determines the reading frame of the mRNA, that is, the three-nucleotide sequence in which mRNA will be read. The ribosome moves in a 5′ to 3′ direction to the next three-nucleotide codon and samples the available tRNAs to find one that matches the mRNA codon. This tRNA transiently binds to the mRNA site via its anticodon. The amino acid from the preceding tRNA (methionine at the beginning) is cleaved and transferred by an enzyme to the amino acid at the end of the new tRNA, forming a new linkage with the carboxyl terminal of the nascent peptide. The ribosome moves another three nucleotides to the next codon and the process is repeated, with the growing chain of amino acids each time being transferred to

THE GENETIC CODE

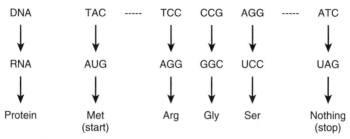

FIGURE 1–9. **The Central Dogma: DNA to RNA to Protein, in Code.** The figure shows the three-letter code in DNA and the complementary code in RNA with U (uridine) substituting for T (thymidine). AUG calls for methionine and the start of translation. UAG and, in addition, UAA and AGA call for no amino acid and the end of translation.

the incoming tRNA. Thus the mRNA provides the code, the ribosome facilitates, and the tRNA is the vehicle for growth of the peptide chain.

Termination of translation, the end of the peptide chain, is not positively signaled, rather it results from the lack of a signal. When the mRNA codon represents no amino acid, no new tRNA appears, hydrolysis of the peptidyl-tRNA occurs, the completed peptide is released from the last tRNA, and the ribosomal subunits dissociate. Translation has terminated; the protein backbone has been formed.

# Final Steps in Making the Protein: Post-translational Processing

While amino acids are added in a linear fashion to produce the primary structure of proteins, these proteins assume a secondary and tertiary structure based in part on the interaction of the component amino acids. The tertiary structure of proteins determines their chemistry and functions; for example, enzymes form binding pockets for substrates, and receptors make sites for selective binding of ligands.

Proteins fold into their correct shape as a result of the polar nature of amino acids. Polar or hydrophobic amino acids tend to be pushed to the center of proteins to avoid contact with water, whereas nonpolar amino acids appear at the outside of proteins to interact with water. Bonding between amino acids provides weak hydrogen-mediated *noncovalent bonds*, or strong *covalent* charge-related bonds that hold the protein in its folded structure. The folded proteins assume the shape of sheets; their secondary structure and these sheets then interact to form domains. *Structural motifs* refer to commonly shared tertiary structures that the folded sheets assume. The folding process is not a simple function of amino acid charge interactions

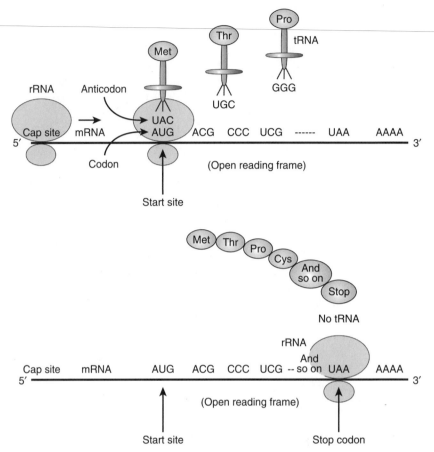

FIGURE 1–10. **Translation: Putting rRNA and tRNA to Work.** Once mRNA is transported to the cytoplasm, it associates with ribosomal RNA (rRNA) at the mRNA cap site. rRNA then scans the mRNA in a 5′ to 3′ direction, locking on to mRNA at AUG, the methionine codon that signifies the translation start site. rRNA then acts as a docking site for transfer RNA (tRNA), which carries the amino acids to the nascent (forming) peptide chain. There is a different tRNA for each amino acid. At the end opposite the amino acid is an anticodon that is complementary to the mRNA codon for the amino acid. The tRNA docks at AUG and translation begins; methionine starts the chain. A second tRNA with its amino acid docks at the next codon and a peptide bond forms between the two amino acids, in this case methionine and threonine, leaving the first tRNA free to move from the ribosome. rRNA moves down the mRNA one codon at a time. New tRNAs bring their amino acids to the growing peptide chain until a codon such as UAA is encountered. Since no tRNA will recognize the UAA codon, the ribosome releases from mRNA and synthesis of the peptide is ended.

because the timing and cellular site of protein folding must also be controlled. A growing number of molecules called chaperones have been described that appear to regulate the folding process.

Post-translational processing of proteins involves the folding process that determines structure and function, but it also involves targeting of protein to the proper site in the cell and the addition of sugars to the peptide chains. Proteins are of two types, those that contain a signal peptide, directing the protein to the ER, and those that do not. The ER is a large perinuclear collection of membranes that form tubules into which ribosomes with nascent proteins are transported. Proteins destined to be transported to the cell membrane for insertion or secretion or proteins to be retained in the ER are processed in the ER (Fig. 1–11). The processing of proteins in the ER and Golgi apparatus are discussed further in Chapters 5 and 6. Proteins are further processed by the addition of sugar side chains (glycosylation); by phosphorylation (activation); or by dephosphorylation of serine, threonine, or tyrosine residues as well as by cross-linking in the extracellular space; they are degraded at various rates. All these events are included under the term post-translational processing. Each is important in determining protein abundance, protein structure, and protein function.

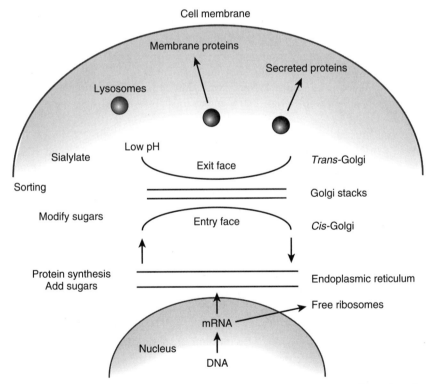

FIGURE 1–11. **Post-translational Processing of Proteins.** Proteins are synthesized on free ribosomes in the cytoplasm and are transferred to the endoplasmic reticulum (ER), where they are partially glycosylated. Some return to the ER and nucleus and others enter the Golgi apparatus, where they are further modified and are sorted for transport back to the ER or nucleus or are targeted in the *trans*-Golgi for degradation in lysosomes, for secretion, or for insertion into the cell membrane.

## Molecular Geography: Measuring DNA, RNA, and Protein

The techniques most commonly used to identify and quantify DNA, RNA, and proteins share several features in common: (1) isolation of the molecular species of interest; (2) separation of the DNA, RNA, or protein by size (migration in an electrical field); (3) transfer of separated material to some type of filter; and (4) probing the filter with a molecule that binds to a specific DNA, RNA, or protein and can itself provide a signal that can be recognized and quantified.

Each of the major methods for recognizing these molecules has a geographic title. Measurement of DNA by this approach is the Southern method or *Southern blot*, named after its inventor; RNA is analyzed by the *Northern blot*; and protein is analyzed by the *Western blot*. It should come as no surprise that identification of a protein transcription factor bound to a segment of DNA using these methods is a *Southwestern blot*. So far there is no Eastern blot.

Whole organisms, organs, tissues, or cells can serve as the source of DNA, RNA, or protein. DNA is stable and has been successfully extracted from prehistoric plants and animals. DNA is the same in all somatic (nonsex) cells, so the source of DNA does not matter. The DNA extracted from brain or lung is the same as that extracted from skin cells or circulating leukocytes. RNA is much less stable than DNA and it must be worked with carefully in the laboratory; for example, human hands have RNAse on them, thus gloves are worn and glassware is specially prepared for RNA work. The RNA of greatest interest is mRNA, which represents only 1% to 5% of total RNA. The other RNAs (rRNA and tRNA) tend to be constitutively expressed and are not organ- or cell-specific, nor do they tell us much about the rates of gene transcription. mRNA represents only those DNA molecules that are transcribed and processed at a particular time and in a particular cell. For example, the lung is the only organ and the type 2 cell the only cell in the body that expresses the mRNA for SPC. Translated protein is obviously also often different in each tissue and cell.

Figure 1–12 outlines the basic processes involved in isolating and measuring DNA, mRNA, and protein. Increasingly, kits and single-step packaged solutions have become available to simplify the extraction process. In general, for isolation of nucleic acids cells or tissues are lysed and DNA or RNA is specifically isolated by any one of a number of methods. DNA is precipitated and cut into manageable pieces with restriction enzymes (see Chapter 2). For total RNA, guanidinium is most frequently used to lyse cells and denature proteins. RNA is separated by centrifugation and is solubilized and precipitated by ethanol. To selectively isolate mRNA, total RNA is passed over a cellulose column to which many thymidine nucleic acids have been immobilized. mRNA almost always has a poly A tail at its 3′ end. The adenines in the poly A tail bind in a complementary fashion to the thymidines of the

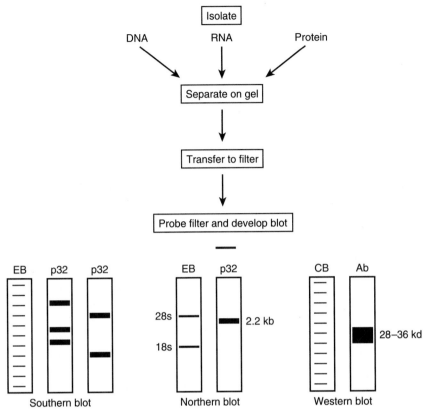

FIGURE 1–12. **Analyzing DNA, RNA, and Proteins: Molecular Geography.** To analyze the amount and structure of DNA, RNA, or protein, they are isolated as described in the text, separated by size in an electrical field on a gel, and transferred to a piece of filter paper. DNA may be cut by a number of different restriction enzymes prior to separation. The filters are then hybridized with a radioactive probe that binds to DNA or RNA as a result of being complementary. The protein gel is incubated with an antibody (Ab) to the protein of interest that has been labeled or can be recognized with a second antibody. EB, ethidium bromide, which binds to nucleic acids; CB, comassie blue, a dye that stains proteins.

column, whereas other RNA types run through. The mRNA is then dissociated from the column and the mRNA is collected by ethanol precipitation. Protein is simply collected by precipitation of the total cell extract.

The RNA, DNA, or protein is separated on the basis of size by electrophoresis; larger species migrate more slowly in the electrical field and distribute at the top of the gel and smaller species migrate to the bottom of the gel. Nucleic acids and proteins are then transferred to some type of filter (usually made of nylon), which can be handled more easily than the gel. In the case of DNA, the gel must first be incubated in alkali to convert double- to single-stranded DNA. Nucleic acids are first immobilized on the filter by baking or exposing the filter to ultraviolet light. The filter is then incubated with a probe that will hybridize to the DNA or RNA by virtue of its complementarity or to protein by nature of its affinity. The keys to recognition of individual molecules are specificity and affinity. If the probes are specific, that is, are chosen to recognize specific nucleotide sequences or specific proteins, the amount (abundance) or the size of a single DNA or mRNA or protein molecule is revealed. Nucleic acid probes must be complementary in order to hybridize. For example, single-stranded cDNA, cRNA, or a string of synthetic nucleotides (oligonucleotides) can be used to probe a Southern blot or Northern blot. The probe must have a tag, usually a radioisotope, which allows it to be recognized, although nonradioactive tags are being used with increasing frequency. The specificity of the interaction between probe and target is defined by stringency conditions. Under low-stringency conditions, hybridization to partially complementary sequences can occur; for example, only 18 of 20 nucleotides need to match. Thus a probe may hybridize to both an exact and related copies of RNA or DNA. Under high-stringency conditions, a probe will hybridize only to perfectly matched sequences, that is, only to an exact complementary copy of RNA or DNA. Stringency is controlled by both temperature and salt conditions during the hybridization reaction or during the subsequent washing of the probed blot. Stringency is increased, made more specific, by raising the temperature and lowering the salt concentration of the incubation or washing solution. This "trick" of modulating specificity of hybridization provides a molecular method that can be used to find conserved, similar but not identical genes in other species that have been conserved throughout evolution, for screening DNA libraries for genes related but not identical to the probe, or for site-directed mutagenesis. Proteins can be recognized by antibodies. Antibodies are either *monoclonal*, that is, derived from a single clone of immunized cells recognizing only a single part of a protein (a single epitope), or *polyclonal*, derived from many cells and recognizing a number of epitopes in a protein. The antibodies can carry a radioisotope tag or may contain a chemical tag that is recognized by a second antibody.

Southern, Northern, and Western blots can provide information about a single DNA, RNA, or protein species. This information can relate to amount, size, or the processed structure of the molecule of interest. The general structure of DNA can be determined by the patterns on a Southern blot created by digestion of DNA with various restriction enzymes (a restriction map of DNA). Isolating and measuring the amount of a specific mRNA in a tissue or cell provides information about what genes are being expressed and at what level or what effect a hormone or growth factor or treatment might have on the expression of a specific gene. In the end, it is proteins that do the work and it is the post-translational processing of proteins that is the last step in the journey from gene to function.

## SUGGESTED READING

Alberts B, Bray D, Lewis J, et al: Molecular Biology of the Cell, 3rd ed. New York, Garland, 1994.

Leder P, Clayton DA, Rubenstein E (eds): Introduction to Molecular Medicine. New York, Scientific American, 1994.

Lewin B: Genes. V. Oxford, Oxford University Press, 1994.

Lodish H, Baltimore D, Berk A, et al: Molecular Cell Biology, 3rd ed. New York, Scientific American Books, W. H. Freeman, 1995.

Rosenfeld N: Molecular medicine. Tools of the trade—recombinant DNA. N Engl J Med 331:315–317, 1994.

Rosenfeld N: Stalking the gene. DNA libraries. N Engl J Med 331:599–600, 1994.

Rosenfeld N: Regulation of gene expression. N Engl J Med 331:931–933, 1994.

Rosenfeld N: Fine structure of a gene—DNA sequencing. N Engl J Med 332:589–591, 1994.

Watson JD, Gilman M, Witkowski J, et al: Recombinant DNA, 2nd ed. New York, Scientific American Books, W.H. Freeman, 1992.

# Tuberculosis

polymerase chain reaction •

DNA fingerprints • restriction enzymes •

restriction fragment length polymorphisms •

insertion elements • DNA libraries •

transfection • vectors • reporter genes •

cloning • single-strand conformational

polymorphism

According to the World Health Organization, infections are the greatest cause of death in the world and tuberculosis (TB) is the leading cause of death due to infections. Each year there are 8 million new cases of TB in the world and 2.9 million deaths from TB (Table 2–1). The World Health Organization projects that there will be 4 million deaths per year from tuberculosis by the year 2005. Approximately one third of the world's population harbors *Mycobacterium tuberculosis*. It is clear that TB in the United States is a small public health problem compared with its impact on developing countries, but a recent change in its incidence in the United States has generated new interest in the basic science of this old disease. There has been a dramatic reversal of the downward trend in TB case rates in the United States over the past several years. During this century, there was a continual decrease in the number of reported new cases of TB until the mid-1980s. Between 1985 and 1991, new cases of TB increased by 18% nationwide. The advent of

TABLE 2–1
**Estimated Annual Tuberculosis Statistics 1985–1990**

| Geographic Area | Annual Risk | New Cases/Year | Deaths/Year |
| --- | --- | --- | --- |
| Africa | 1.5–2.5% | 1,313,000 | 586,000 |
| North Africa | 0.5–1.5% | 323,000 | 91,000 |
| Asia | 1.0–2.0% | 5,102,000 | 1,825,000 |
| South America | 0.5–1.5% | 356,000 | 111,000 |
| Central America | 0.5–1.5% | 185,000 | 80,000 |
| **United States** | **0.02%** | **25,700** | **2,000** |
| World | | 8,000,000 | 2,900,000 |

AIDS and the worldwide recession that resulted in increasing numbers of homeless individuals, along with immigration trends, contributed to the dramatic increase of new TB cases in the United States (approximately 52,000 more cases than predicted).

This resurgence of TB as a public health hazard has generated considerable new interest in the basic science of TB and in particular the application of molecular biologic techniques to the diagnosis and treatment of TB. Four recent advances are presented here because they illustrate specific molecular biologic methods. They deal with new and more rapid approaches to the diagnosis of TB using the polymerase chain reaction (PCR), new approaches to defining the epidemiology of TB using a technique called DNA fingerprinting or restriction fragment length polymorphisms (RFLPs), new ways of diagnosing mycobacterial drug resistance, and attempts to understand the basis of mycobacterial drug resistance. The latter two examples introduce concepts such as DNA libraries, transfection, reporter genes, vectors, gene cloning, and single-strand conformational polymorphisms. Some of the results of these studies have made their way into clinical practice, whereas some are still in developmental stages.

## Rapid Diagnosis: The Polymerase Chain Reaction

Traditionally the diagnosis of TB rests in either finding acid-fast organisms on microscopic examination of smears of sputum or other secretions or in culturing mycobacteria from these specimens. Analysis of smears is rapid and inexpensive but insensitive, requiring more than 100,000 organisms/mL of sample for a positive result (Table 2–2). Culturing mycobacteria is orders of magnitude more sensitive, requiring only 1000 organisms/mL, but cultures take from 2 to 8 weeks to provide positive results. PCR is rapid (less than 24 hours) and extremely sensitive, theoretically requiring as few as two organisms

TABLE 2–2
*Diagnosis of Tuberculosis*

| | Smear | Culture | Probe° | Polymerase Chain Reaction |
|---|---|---|---|---|
| Sensitivity | Very Low | Low | Medium | **High** |
| Speed | Minutes | Weeks | Days | **Hours** |
| Species | No | Yes | Yes | **Yes** |
| % Positive | 20% | 60% | ?? | **100%** |

°The probe method was a *Mycobacterium tuberculosis*–specific probe to perform a Northern blot for *M. tuberculosis* mRNA. It requires more organisms than does PCR.

in a sample. The technique is relatively simple and, once equipment is purchased, inexpensive. However, the exquisite sensitivity of PCR also leads to a number of false-positive and false-negative results, so PCR must be performed under carefully controlled conditions. In addition, PCR indicates the presence of DNA in live or dead organisms; however, it is not an indicator of active infection.

PCR was invented in 1986 and is already used in many clinical settings and as a standard tool in many molecular biologic studies. It has won its inventor, Kerry Mullis, much fame and a Nobel Prize. PCR is a way of amplifying *minute amounts of unique segments of DNA;* it is *sensitive* and *specific.* It is also *simple* and *rapid.* Extraction of DNA and its amplification and identification can be accomplished in less than 24 hours. PCR has been used to study DNA from almost anywhere for anything; virtually any type of sample, from fresh to fossilized, has been analyzed for diagnostic, genetic, forensic, and myriad other purposes (Table 2–3).

PCR requires only a *source of DNA* (in the case of this discussion mycobacteria from sputum, blood, cerebrospinal or pleural fluid, or other

TABLE 2–3
*Analysis by Polymerase Chain Reaction*

| Source of DNA or RNA | Purpose |
|---|---|
| Secretion | Medical diagnosis |
| Cells | Genetics |
| Tissues | Mutations |
| Histologic specimens | Forensics |
| Fossils | Anthropologic studies |
| General | Molecular methods—cloning, sequencing, and so on |

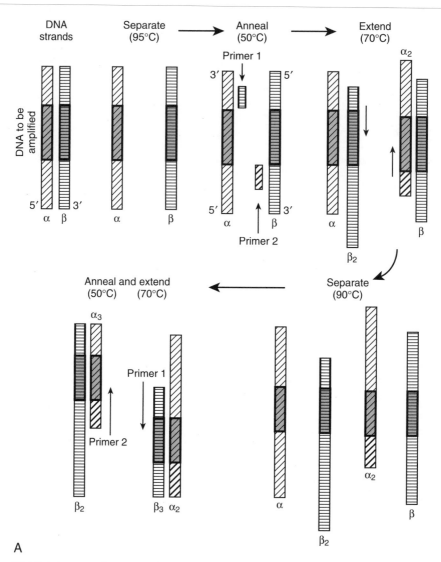

FIGURE 2–1. **A. Polymerase chain reaction (PCR): The Method.** A specific and unique DNA sequence is chosen for the PCR reaction. PCR primers are constructed by synthesizing oligonucleotides that are complementary to the 3' or 5' ends of opposite strands of the piece of DNA to be amplified (*primer 1, primer 2*). The DNA strands are then separated by heating the mixture of DNA, primers, nucleic acids, and the Taq DNA polymerase. The primers anneal (hybridize) to the DNA template at a lower temperature, and the mixture is reheated to allow the DNA polymerase to synthesize DNA in a 3' to 5' direction on each strand. The process is repeated 20 to 40 times, with each cycle increasing the amplified DNA in a logarithmic fashion.

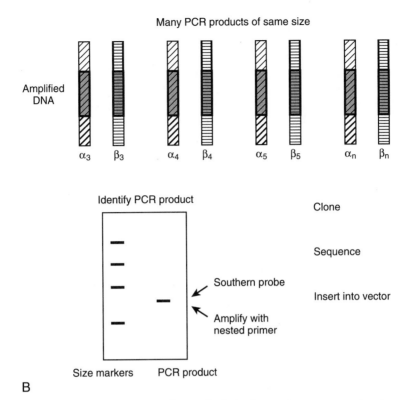

**Many PCR products of same size**

Amplified DNA

$\alpha_3$  $\beta_3$    $\alpha_4$  $\beta_4$    $\alpha_5$  $\beta_5$    $\alpha_n$  $\beta_n$

Identify PCR product

Clone

Sequence

Southern probe

Insert into vector

Amplify with nested primer

Size markers    PCR product

B

FIGURE 2–1 *Continued*. **B. PCR: The Method.** As the reactions progress, the pieces of amplified DNA that accumulate are of the same size, defined by the original design of the primers. The products are identified by running them out on a gel to determine if they are the size predicted by the original primers. The DNA may also be identified by using an internal oligonucleotide (i.e., a probe complementary to some part of the product) in a Southern blot reaction or by designing new internal oligonucleotides (called nested primers) to reamplify the product. The amplified material can be cloned, sequenced, inserted into a vector for transfection, and used for diagnosis or a large number of other purposes.

sources); *oligonucleotide primers*, specifically designed to recognize unique sequences of the target DNA; a source of the basic building blocks of DNA, *deoxynucleotide triphosphates;* a *DNA polymerase* that is not denatured at high temperature; and some type of *thermocycling device* that alters the temperature of the reaction mixture in a programmable fashion. The heat-resistant DNA polymerase comes from an aquatic bacterium *(Thermus aquaticus)* found in hot springs and is commonly called Taq polymerase.

The primers are chosen to match a base sequence at the 3′ end of each strand of DNA to be amplified (Fig. 2–1A). The primers are in the range of 20 oligonucleotides (called a 20 mer). The combination of two sets of bases of this length have a $10^{20}$ chance of binding to an unrelated piece of DNA. Thus, there is virtually no chance of the two primers hybridizing or annealing to and amplifying an unrelated stretch of DNA because there are only $10^9$ bases in the human genome and fewer in the mycobacterial genome. Of importance is the fact that the primers that bind to each strand of DNA are complementary to that portion of DNA, and therefore they are identical to the DNA on the opposite strand.

The principle of PCR is illustrated in Figures 2–1A and 2–1B. The process involves repetitive cycles of alternating temperatures that result in (1) separation of the two DNA strands, (2) annealing specific primers to the individual strands, and (3) synthesizing two new strands of DNA. In Figure 2–1, the two strands of DNA ($\alpha$ and $\beta$) are shown, with the area of DNA that will be amplified on complementary strands shaded. This area should be one that is unique to the target gene of interest. The thermocyler is then heated to 95°C to separate the two DNA strands, and the temperature is lowered to allow the oligonucleotide primers *(primer 1 and primer 2)* to anneal or bind to the 3′ end of each DNA strand. Once the synthetic oligonucleotides have annealed, the temperature is raised again, this time to the 70°C range, and the DNA polymerase goes to work, using the deoxy-nucleotide substrate to synthesize or extend each new complementary DNA strand in a 3′ to 5′ direction. The cycle is then repeated, heating to break apart the newly synthesized strands, annealing the primers to both old and new strands, and extending the strands again. In this cycle, primer 1 anneals to the 3′ end of the newly synthesized $\beta_2$ strand, and primer 2 anneals to the 3′ end of the newly synthesized $\alpha_2$ strand, and the process of extension is repeated. As primers anneal to new strands, the size of each of the new complementary strands is defined as the distance between the two primers (see Fig. 2–2). Since the number of strands doubles after each cycle, DNA is amplified in an exponential fashion. Thus, after 30 cycles there are $2^{30}$ DNA strands, virtually all of them being of the size determined by the distance between the two primers. The DNA can then be run out on a gel, and the identity of the reaction products can be confirmed either by the predicted size of new DNA or with a Southern blot, probing the DNA in the gel with an oligonucleotide that recognizes some internal sequence in the amplified DNA, or by repeating the PCR reaction using a new set of specific primers (nested primers) that recognize sequences within the amplified DNA. The amplified segment can be used for the diagnosis of *M. tuberculosis* in this example, or the piece of DNA can be cloned, sequenced, inserted into a vector, and transfected into another cell.

PCR can amplify artifacts such as DNA contaminants, but these contaminants are not of the predicted size nor are they recognized by internal oligonucleotides. A number of positive and negative controls must be run with each reaction to ensure that all the reagents are functional. However, with appropriate concerns about false-positive and false-negative results, PCR has become an extremely powerful tool for recognizing specific DNA sequences in a variety of samples. As noted in Table 2–3, this method can be applied to DNA or RNA (the RNA is reverse transcribed into DNA) obtained from secretions, blood, cells, virtually any tissue, and paraffin-embedded histologic specimens. In addition, because DNA is a stable molecule, PCR can be applied to bones and fossils that are millions of years old. Indeed, a recent study of ancient human bones has shown that *M. tuberculosis* was the cause of Pott's disease more than 1000 years ago. The number of clinical applications continues to increase, as do the number of applications to new molecular biologic techniques.

The first requirement for using PCR to diagnose TB is a gene that is unique to TB, that is, not shared by any other organisms. Until recently, suprisingly little information was available about proteins that are produced by *M. tuberculosis*. Indeed, little of the *M. tuberculosis* genome has been sequenced, and this has become a major focus of investigators in the field. A recent cooperative study compiled a list of mycobacteria antigens, most of which have been described in the last several years. Some of the better characterized antigens are heat shock proteins, some are secreted with uncertain function, some are lipoproteins, and one is a superoxide dismutase.

PCR studies have focused on genes coding for proteins that are exclusively expressed in organisms of the *M. tuberculosis* complex, which includes *M. tuberculosis* and *M. bovis* but not *M. kansasii* or *M. avium*. It is possible to find genes that are expressed in all mycobacteria species or genes that differ sufficiently to be able to allow identification of individual species. It is clear that the primers one uses for PCR diagnosis of TB should be chosen on the basis of what species of mycobacteria one is looking for. The ideal gene should also be expressed in high copy number, that is, the gene should be abundant in the mycobacteria genome rather than rare because the more abundant the genes, the more sensitive the test will be. At present, most studies are performed with an *M. tuberculosis* complex–specific insertion element (see later discussion of DNA fingerprinting for further discussion of this element).

Because of its potential for rapid and sensitive diagnosis of *M. tuberculosis*, there have been a large number of studies published in the past few years that applied PCR methods to diagnose TB. The results to date suggest that PCR is a highly sensitive, specific test with strong positive and negative predictability for active tuberculosis. The value of the test depends in part on the patient population one is studying. PCR recognizes mycobacterial DNA; it does not determine whether the mycobacteria are alive or are part of an active infection. Thus, performing PCR on tissue, sputum, or bronchoscopic specimens from patients who have had prior treated or untreated TB that is now inactive may yield a number of false-positive results. PCR produces positive results on the DNA of dormant (noninfectious) bacteria. Despite this drawback, the results of most studies have been surprisingly similar. PCR produces close to 100% positive results in individuals with positive smear results and greater than 90% positive results in patients with negative smear results but positive culture results. PCR results are also positive in some individuals with negative smear and culture results but whose subsequent clinical course is suggestive of active disease.

At present, methods of treating specimens, isolating DNA, choosing genes to amplify, designing appropriate oligonucleotide primers, including negative and positive controls, and verifying results are being tested and standardized, and commercial kits are available. However, the simplicity, sensitivity, and rapidity of the procedure ensure that PCR will become one of the standard methods for diagnosing TB in the future. Because one can design primers that are species-specific, PCR also holds promise as a rapid way of typing TB organisms and ultimately in determining patterns of specific drug resistance.

PCR has also been applied to sputum samples and bronchoalveolar lavage for the diagnosis of *Pneumocystis carinii* pneumonia, cytomegalovirus, and *Mycoplasma* pneumonia, as well as other fungal pathogens. The results are similar to those with *M. tuberculosis*, although many of these organisms are normal respiratory tract inhabitants; therefore, finding the organism does not establish the presence of active infection. Recently, performing PCR on white blood cells in circulating blood for some of these organisms and for *M. tuberculosis* has proved to be a rapid and reliable way of diagnosing active infection.

## DNA Fingerprinting: New Epidemiologic Tools that Use Restriction Endonucleases

As noted earlier, the resurgence of TB as a public health hazard, particularly in patients with human immunodeficiency virus (HIV) disease, has raised concerns about patterns of transmission and ways of charting its spread in high-risk patients. The question of whether the increased incidence of TB in HIV-infected patients is a consequence of altered immunity and breakdown of endogenous infection or increased susceptibility to exogenous infection is also of concern. In the past, phage typing was the only epidemiologic tool for identifying different TB isolates. However, this is a time-consuming method that has limited ability to distinguish among TB isolates.

The molecular technique of DNA fingerprinting has recently been applied to this problem and has produced important new observations. A number of studies have established these methods as extremely effective tools that have great potential in the clinical epidemiology of TB. This subject also provides an opportunity to present important molecular methods and concepts such as restriction enzymes, RFLPs, and insertion elements.

Restriction endonucleases are invaluable for a number of molecular methods, including cloning, DNA sequencing, transgenic technology, RFLPs, and DNA fingerprinting. In the 1970s, it was discovered that bacteria contained nuclear DNA cutting enzymes. The enzymes were called restriction enzymes because they restricted the entry of foreign DNA into bacteria by cleaving it at specific sites (restriction sites). These enzymes do not cut DNA in a random fashion; rather, they recognize specific nucleotide sequences that range from four to eight base pairs in length. Enzymes that recognize short nucleotide sequences cut DNA frequently, producing many small pieces. Enzymes that recognize longer sequences are rare DNA cutters producing fewer but larger pieces of DNA. Figure 2–2 shows that some enzymes, such as Hae III, make straight cuts between strands, whereas some, such as EcoRI, make jagged cuts between strands. The type of cut influences how "sticky" the ends of the cut DNA are, a point that is discussed further on in the section on cloning. There are currently so many restriction enzymes available (>200), each recognizing and cutting specific nucleotide sequences, that one can choose the point at which to cut DNA to create precise pieces of DNA that can be used for specific purposes.

Once cut, by one or a combination of several restriction enzymes, the DNA pieces can be separated by size by electrophoresis in an agarose gel (see Chapter 1). By staining the gel with a dye that binds to DNA (e.g., ethidium bromide), the various DNA fragments can be recognized. Different enzymes produce different pieces of DNA. The restriction digest patterns depend on the frequency of enzyme recognition sites within the DNA of interest.

*Polymorphisms*, meaning many forms, are differences in DNA sequences that result from mutations. Changes in sequence have the potential of altering the patterns of restriction enzyme cutting of DNA. Although some changes in restriction fragments can be seen on agarose gels stained for DNA, the

Restriction enzymes and their cleavage sequences
(>200 enzymes described)

| Organism | Enzyme | Sequence |
|----------|--------|----------|
| *Haemophilus aegyptius* | Hae III | 5'..........G G\|C C..........3'<br>3'..........C C\|G G..........3' |
| *Escherichia coli* | EcoR I | 5'........G\|A A T T C........3'<br>3'........C T T A A\|G.......5' |
| *N. otitidis* | Not I | 5'...G\|C G G C C G C...3'<br>3'...C G C C G G C\|G...5' |

FIGURE 2–2. **Restriction Enzymes and Their Cleavage Sites.** Bacterial DNA cutting enzymes recognize specific sequences of nucleotides and cut the DNA at the places indicated. These cuts are either blunt-ended, as is the case for Hae III, or jagged, as is the case for the other two enzymes. Some enzymes are frequent cutters with recognition sequences of only four bases; others are rare cutters (Not I) that recognize only a continuous sequence of eight bases. This long recognition sequence appears relatively infrequently, and therefore the DNA is cut into large pieces.

analysis of RFLPs can be much more sensitive and specific if one uses a DNA probe that recognizes the site included or excluded from a restriction fragment.

It seems reasonable that the genome of mycobacteria of the *M. tuberculosis* complex differs from that of nontuberculous mycobacteria and therefore that their RFLPs will differ. However, differences among individual isolates of the *M. tuberculosis* complex are likely to be more subtle. This is where insertion elements come into the picture. Insertion elements are short DNA sequences that can move from one place in the bacterial genome to another and can actually undergo duplication in a new site. Insertion sequences (IS) are found in different places in the genome of different strains of bacterial organisms. Insertion sequences have no known function but are widely distributed in bacteria. They generally do not encode proteins, so unless they are inserted to interfere with gene function they are silent markers that can be used to distinguish one bacterial strain from another.

The insertion sequence IS6110 has been found in *M. tuberculosis* complex organisms; it occurs in multiple copies in *M. tuberculosis* and as a single copy, or at least fewer copies, in *M. bovis*. It has not been found in other mycobacteria. Several recent studies have combined the restriction enzyme–RFLP approach with IS6110 used as a DNA probe to develop a new epidemiologic tool called DNA fingerprinting.

Genomic DNA is extracted from the patient's TB culture, and the DNA is cut with any one of a number of restriction enzymes (Fig. 2–3). The DNA is then separated by size in an agarose gel as with RFLP analysis, after which the DNA is transferred to a piece of filter paper with a charged surface to which the DNA tightly binds as in the Southern blots described in Chapter 1. The filter with the transferred DNA is then incubated (hybridized) with a IS6110 cDNA probe that has been tagged with phosphorus-32. The IS6110 cDNA is complementary to the IS6110 sequence in the *M. tuberculosis* DNA and therefore binds tightly and specifically to *M. tuberculosis* IS6110 wherever it is on the gel. This hybridization is so tight that the probe cannot be washed off the filter. The filter is then exposed to film and an autoradiograph shows to which pieces of DNA the IS6110 probe has bound. This process produces a unique profile for each set of mycobacterial organisms.

The epidemiologic power of this method has been shown in tracing epidemics to source cases. It is now clear that mycobacteria retain the same DNA fingerprints for long periods, both in vitro and in vivo during a relapse. In addition, the fingerprints do not appear to change when drug resistance is induced in vitro. Two recent studies have used DNA fingerprinting to analyze transmission patterns of TB in New York City and in San Francisco. All positive culture results were fingerprinted using restriction digests of mycobacterial DNA probed with the IS6110 insertion element. Despite the different populations of subjects, the two studies came to surprisingly similar conclusions by combining fingerprints with standard epidemiologic techniques. They both found that at least 30 to 40% of new cases were due to

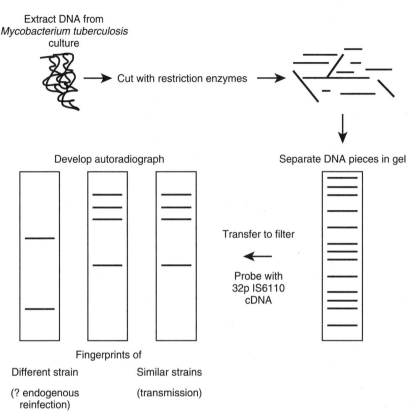

Extract DNA from
*Mycobacterium tuberculosis*
culture

→ Cut with restriction enzymes →

Separate DNA pieces in gel

Transfer to filter
←
Probe with
32p IS6110
cDNA

Develop autoradiograph

Fingerprints of

Different strain

(? endogenous
reinfection)

Similar strains

(transmission)

FIGURE 2–3. **DNA Fingerprinting.** Genomic DNA is extracted from cultures of *Mycobacterium tuberculosis* and cut with restriction enzymes; the resultant pieces are separated by size in a gel. The DNA is transferred to filter paper, which is then incubated (hybridized) with a radioactive probe that is complementary to the insertion element IS6110 (see text). This element inserts at random places in the *M. tuberculosis* genome but remains at the same place over time in each *M. tuberculosis* isolate. Therefore, IS6110 patterns characterize transmission patterns of *M. tuberculosis* within populations. Individuals with the same fingerprint are infected with the same organism, which was likely transmitted from the same source case. Individuals with different fingerprints have different source cases. Unique fingerprints are likely the result of endogenous breakdown of pre-existing bacterial foci rather than recent transmission of new bacteria.

recent person-to-person transmission rather than reactivation of latent infection. In HIV-infected individuals, almost two thirds of patients had evidence of recent transmission rather than reactivation of latent infection. In foreign-born individuals, the fingerprints suggested that the predominant cause of newly diagnosed active tuberculosis was reactivation of latent TB rather than person-to-person transmission. These findings have begun to alter public health approaches to the management of tuberculosis. Thus, the epidemiologic power of the TB DNA fingerprint method is obvious, although the lack of IS6110 in mycobacteria other than those of the *M. tuberculosis* complex does limit the application of this method somewhat.

As is the case with the PCR methods discussed previously, a collaborative approach to the use of restriction enzymes and standardization of methods seems appropriate so that the methods can be used to gather worldwide information about disease transmission patterns. It also seems clear that this method will help in the diagnosis of drug-resistant mycobacterial disease. If individuals have mycobacterial DNA fingerprints that are identical to those of a patient with known drug-resistant disease, they can be presumed to have drug-resistant TB also.

A similar approach is involved in the DNA fingerprinting used in forensic medicine. In this case, the DNA probe includes one of several variable numbers of tandemly repeated units that are randomly distributed in genomic DNA and distinguish one individual from another. For DNA fingerprints, DNA is extracted from virtually any source of tissues or cells and digested with restriction enzymes, separated on a gel, and hybridized with probes for each variable number of a tandemly repeated unit. The resultant RFLPs have become important legal tests in establishing paternity and in identifying blood, skin, semen, or hair samples. Estimates are that the chances of random identity between DNA from the subject in question and that of the sample range between $1 \times 10^5$ and $1 \times 10^6$.

## Reporter Genes Shed Light on Mycobacterial Drug Resistance

Because *M. tuberculosis* is such a slowly growing organism, it usually takes weeks or months to produce enough organisms to determine to which drugs the patient's organisms are sensitive. This has led to the practice of treating high-risk patients with four or more often toxic drugs until drug-resistance studies have been completed many weeks later. A recently published method using molecular techniques promises a new, rapid test of drug resistance that will provide information on fewer organisms (perhaps as few as 100) in as little as 2 to 3 days. Although many details must be worked out before it is applied clinically, this test provides an opportunity to discuss reporter genes and methods of introducing foreign DNA into cells or organisms.

Reporter genes are used in a variety of molecular experiments to indicate the presence and magnitude of a reaction. The discussion of gene regulation in Chapter 8 illustrates how reporters such as chloramphenicol transferase and human growth hormone have been used to define active regulatory elements in the surfactant genes. Firefly luciferase has become a popular reporter gene because of its sensitivity and ease of measurement. In the firefly, luciferase catalyzes the oxidation of luciferin in the presence of an energy source—adenosine triphosphate (ATP), producing light (Fig. 2–4). Used as a reporter, the reaction is a quantitative measure of ATP availability and requires only a sensitive light-detection system. Since firefly luciferase cDNA has been cloned, it can be transfected (inserted) into any cell, and the

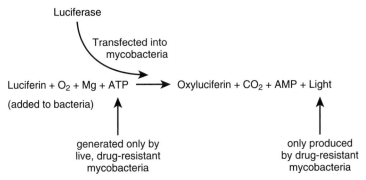

FIGURE 2–4. **Reporter Genes: How the Firefly Makes Light.** In the presence of the exogenous substrate luciferin and adenosine triphosphate (ATP), luciferase catalyzes the production of oxyluciferin, generating light in the process. When excess luciferin is present, the amount of light generated is a direct function of the amount of ATP present. The light produced can be quantitatively measured in a luminometer.

luciferase protein can be expressed in that cell if driven by a strong promoter (a DNA sequence that is recognized by transcription factors that are present in every cell and that supports active transcription, in this case of the luciferase cDNA). When the exogenous substrate luciferin is added to cells expressing luciferase, the amount of light generated by that cell (measured in a fluorometer) is a direct function of the amount of ATP generated by the cell. How does luciferase help diagnose *M. tuberculosis* drug sensitivity? Mycobacteria die in the presence of an antituberculous drug to which they are sensitive. Dead organisms generate little ATP and thus do not produce light when transfected with luciferase and provided with exogenous luciferin (Fig. 2–5). Transfected organisms resistant to anti-TB drugs continue to be metabolically active in the presence of those drugs and continue to generate ATP and therefore produce light in the presence of luciferin. This new test, once modified for general use, promises a simple rapid screening tool for identifying drug-resistant mycobacteria.

Because this test of antibiotic resistance requires transfection of cells with DNA, this might be an appropriate place to discuss how cells are transfected, that is, how foreign DNA is introduced into cells. The transfer of pieces of DNA or whole genes into cells is an important technical tool for gene function studies, gene regulation, and gene therapy. Gene transfer or transfection was first studied in tumor viruses that infect mammalian cells and insert their own genetic material into the recipient cell. There are two important steps in the transfection process; getting DNA into the cell and functional expression of the DNA once it is inside the cell.

The first step involves one of a number of mechanical tricks that move the vector or DNA itself into a cell (Fig. 2–6). *Vectors* are autonomously replicating DNA molecules into which fragments of foreign DNA can be inserted; once transfected, they can propagate within the host cell. Types of

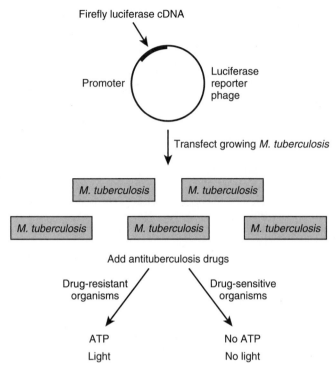

FIGURE 2–5. **Firefly Luciferase Provides a Test for *Mycobacterium tuberculosis* Drug Resistance.** The firefly luciferase cDNA, driven by a strong promoter, is inserted into a phage vector that is capable of transfecting *M. tuberculosis*. If *M. tuberculosis* in culture is transfected with this luciferase construct and then grown in the presence of an antibiotic such as isoniazid (INH) or rifampin, drug-sensitive *M. tuberculosis* will die and produce little ATP and therefore little light, whereas drug-resistant *M. tuberculosis* will continue to produce ATP and light. Theoretically, the amount of light generated can be used to build a drug dose-response curve.

vectors and methods of DNA insertion into vectors will be discussed further on. The most direct means of transferring a DNA vector into a cell is by microinjection into the cell nucleus. This is an effective method; however, it is technically difficult and can be performed with only small numbers of cells. Most other transfection techniques depend on the cell's natural ability to undergo endocytosis, a process that incorporates material on the cell surface into the cell cytoplasm. DNA enters the cell and survives the various degradative cytoplasmic enzymes and is transferred into the nucleus where, under the right circumstances, it is transcribed.

One method of presenting DNA vectors to the cells is to concentrate them at the cell surface. DNA forms a complex with dextran via charge differences, forming aggregates that can be taken up by cells. DNA in a phosphate buffer forms precipitates when calcium chloride is added, and the calcium phosphate precipitates are incorporated into the cell. Lipofection involves *liposomes*, which are artificial lipid vesicles into which DNA can be

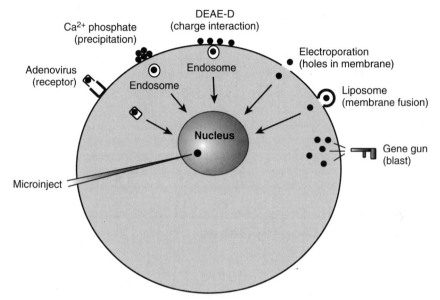

FIGURE 2–6. **Methods of Transfection: Physical, Receptor-Mediated, and Other Methods for Introducing DNA into a Cell.** In each method of transfection, the DNA has to reach the nucleus in order to be transcribed. See text for discussion of each method.

incorporated. These vesicles fuse with cell membranes delivering DNA directly to the cytoplasm, bypassing the endocytic vesicles that often lead to DNA degradation. DNA in solution can be introduced into cells by *electroporation*, in which cells are subject to a brief electrical current that makes transient holes in the cell membrane, allowing DNA to move inside. This technique is particularly useful for cells such as macrophages and lymphocytes, which grow in suspension. Many cells, including difficult to transfect epithelial cells, have receptors for adenoviruses, and adenovirus vectors engineered to eliminate their replicative machinery, or adenovirus mixed with other vectors, have been used to increase endocytosis and the efficiency of transfection. Finally, a new technique called *biolistics* involves coating small gold or tungsten particles with DNA and shooting the particles via compressed air into cells and tissues.

The various transfection methods differ in efficiency and technical complexity. Some cells are easily transfected, whereas others are fragile and are injured during transfection. Some experiments require that only a few cells be successfully transfected, whereas others require that the majority of cells be transfected. There is no single method that is perfect for all cells.

Once in the cell, the vector with its inserted DNA segments must avoid the degradative enzymes of the cytoplasm and make its way into the nucleus, where it is either transiently expressed or stably incorporated into the genetic machinery of the cell. *Transient transfection* is the usual outcome unless an attempt has been made to select those cells that have integrated the transfected DNA into their own genomes and then pass the DNA on to daughter cells during DNA replication. *Stable transfectants* are usually selected by adding a drug resistance gene (usually an antibiotic resistance gene) in the vector, driven by a strong universal promoter. If the antibiotic is added to the medium of the transfected cells, only those cells that have been transfected and express the antibiotic resistance gene survive. This approach results in selection of an antibiotic-resistant cell line that stably expresses the gene of interest.

## Mycobacterial Drug Resistance: Screening Libraries and Cloning Genes

The emergence of drug-resistant forms of mycobacteria has become one of the major problems preventing control of TB in developing countries, among the homeless of American cities, and in HIV-infected individuals. Infection with multidrug-resistant *M. tuberculosis* carries a 70 to 90% mortality rate in HIV patients. Despite the increasing importance of drug resistance, until recently little had been known about the mechanisms of TB drug resistance; indeed little had been known about how anti-TB drugs work. In the past several years, investigators have begun to apply the tools of molecular biology to this important public health problem, and the molecular basis for some forms of isoniazid (INH), rifampin, streptomycin, and pyrazinamide drug resistance have recently been identified (see later).

Two different *M. tuberculosis* mutations have recently been described in INH-resistant *M. tuberculosis*. One mutation affects activation of INH; the other interferes with the binding of activated INH to its target. Both studies defining these mutations have used similar approaches, transferring pieces of genomic DNA from INH-sensitive mycobacteria into INH-resistant mycobacteria or DNA from resistant bacteria into sensitive bacteria and then identifying the DNA that conferred resistance or sensitivity to INH by screening a genomic mycobacterial DNA library. One laboratory has identified loss of catalase activity and a mutation in the *M. tuberculosis* catalase gene *(katG)* as important. Catalase appears to be involved in converting INH to its active form. Between 25 and 50% of INH-resistant isolates display this mutation. Another laboratory has identified a new gene, *InhA*; mutations in the regulatory region of *InhA* have been identified in approximately 25% of resistant organisms. INH and ethionamide are believed to kill mycobacteria by interfering with the synthesis of mycolic acid, a fatty acid that is part of the mycobacterial cell wall. The mutation found in *InhA* prevents INH from blocking mycolic acid synthesis. This discussion focuses on the INH resistance associated with catalase deficiency. It provides an opportunity to introduce a number of fundamental molecular techniques and concepts.

The experiments depicted in Figure 2–7 were carried out in four main stages, each of which illustrates a new molecular biologic concept. The first step in these experiments was to identify a mutant strain of mycobacteria that was highly resistant to INH. Next, genomic DNA was isolated from an INH-sensitive mycobacterial strain, the DNA was cut with restriction enzymes as discussed earlier, and the DNA pieces were packaged in plasmids that could be used to transform INH-resistant organisms. Transformation is a genetic change in bacteria that occurs after exposure to and recombination with DNA from a genetically different bacteria.

*Plasmids* are small circular pieces of bacterial or viral DNA that are capable of independent replication in a host cell. Plasmids and other DNA vectors contain, or can have placed in them, information that allows them not only to survive in host cells but also to function in cells of different species. In this study, a *cosmid*, which is a special type of plasmid vector that accommodates insertion of large pieces of DNA (30,000 base pairs or 30

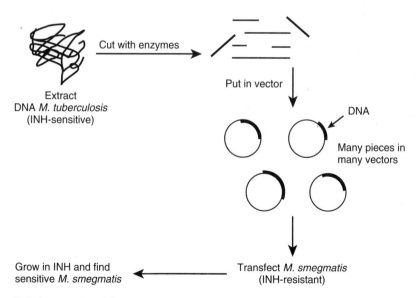

Finding the INH resistance gene

Cut with enzymes

Extract
DNA *M. tuberculosis*
(INH-sensitive)

Put in vector

DNA

Many pieces in
many vectors

Grow in INH and find
sensitive *M. smegmatis*

Transfect *M. smegmatis*
(INH-resistant)

Note increase in catalase

FIGURE 2–7. **Finding the INH Resistance Gene.** DNA from INH-sensitive *M. tuberculosis* is extracted and cut with restriction enzymes and placed in vectors that are then transfected into INH-resistant *M. smegmatis*. Each vector contains a single piece of DNA. Those transfected *M. smegmatis* organisms that become INH-sensitive are noted to increase their catalase activity, suggesting that a piece of DNA related to the catalase gene was involved in conferring sensitivity to INH.

kilobases) to be inserted, was used. The cosmid vector also required additional regulatory information so that it could function in both bacteria and mycobacteria. This type of vector is called a shuttle vector because of its ability to shuttle between the organisms. Some of the cosmids carried DNA from *Escherichia coli* to *M. tuberculosis*, resulting in a change in sensitivity to INH.

Many vectors now commercially available offer features that assist in the cloning and transformation processes (Fig. 2–8). Most vectors contain (1) an origin of replication that allows its efficient replication in the host cells; (2) some means of selecting bacteria that have incorporated and are expressing the vector, such as an antibiotic resistance gene that allows growth of bacteria in the presence of an otherwise lethal antibiotic; (3) a polylinker site that can be cut by any one of a number of different restriction enzymes, allowing insertion of foreign DNA; (4) a variety of constitutive (constant) or inducible

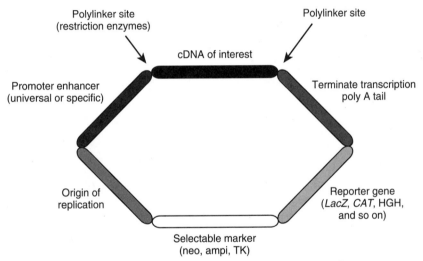

FIGURE 2–8. **Vectors: What Do They Contain and How Do They Work?** Vectors are circular pieces of bacterial or viral DNA that are capable of independent replication in a host cell. To accomplish the independent replication, they contain an origin of replication that drives DNA synthesis. Vectors have a variety of sites that can be cut with restriction enzymes, allowing insertion of the DNA to be transfected. Many vectors now contain polylinker sites that can be cut by a variety of different enzymes. The DNA can be cut by the same enzyme, if it contains such sites, or can have attached to it linkers that have designed restriction sites. The gene of interest can be driven by a strong constitutive promoter—for example, a viral promoter that will result in universal expression—or it can be driven by a cell-specific promoter such as the SPC promoter, which will result in expression only in SPC-expressing cells. Expression vectors designed to produce large amounts of protein contain 3′ structures that stabilize the mRNA and terminate transcription in an efficient fashion. All vectors have some type of selection system that allows only those cells that are transfected to survive. Many vectors contain reporter genes such as luciferase, chloramphenicol transferase, or human growth hormone to indicate the cells or tissues in which the vector is expressed. These positive reporters produce a signal in transfected cells. Another type of reporter system involves insertion of the DNA into the middle of the *LacZ* gene, interrupting transcription of that reporter and resulting in a loss of color in transfected cells.

promoters that drive transcription of inserted DNA; and (5) some sort of reporter gene that marks the cells that are expressing the gene of interest. The *lacZ* gene, which encodes the enzyme β-galactosidase, is used most often. This enzyme turns the exogenous substrate x-gal blue, thereby identifying cells expressing the transfected DNA. Eukaryotic expression vectors are used to express large amounts of the proteins encoded by the gene of interest. These vectors contain, in addition to the components already described, strong universal promoters and enhancers to ensure active transcription of the inserted gene and a poly A tail to stabilize the gene's mRNA so that it can be efficiently translated.

The transformed INH-resistant organisms in the INH resistance experiment were then exposed to INH, and organisms that had become sensitive to INH as a result of transformation with a piece of DNA from the INH-sensitive *M. tuberculosis* were noted to have dramatically increased catalase activity (see Fig. 2–7). It has been known for some time that low catalase activity is a common feature of INH-resistant *M. tuberculosis*. The investigators then used the knowledge that the catalase of *M. tuberculosis* was chemically similar to an enzyme (hydroperoxidase) of *E. coli* and to a similar enzyme in a *Bacillus* organism to design a series of oligonucleotide probes that allowed them to search for and find the *M. tuberculosis* catalase gene in an *M. tuberculosis* genomic DNA library. The probes were constructed by finding amino acid sequences that were similar in the *E. coli* and *Baccillus* proteins and figuring out which of the nucleotides could have coded for these conserved amino acids. The assumption was that if the amino acids were conserved in the two bacterial species, they were likely important for protein function and would be conserved in *M. tuberculosis*. The synthetic oligonucleotide could then be used as a probe to search for the mycobacterial gene that coded for the peroxidase-equivalent gene (catalase) in *M. tuberculosis*.

To find the *M. tuberculosis katG*-equivalent gene, the oligonucleotide probe was used to screen a genomic DNA library of INH-sensitive *M. tuberculosis*. Two types of DNA libraries can be constructed (Fig. 2–9): (1) *genomic libraries* containing all the information within nuclear DNA (regulatory and coding information as well as junk) and (2) *cDNA libraries* that contain only that information that is present in cytoplasmic mRNA (mostly protein coding information). DNA is isolated to construct genomic libraries, whereas mRNA is isolated and converted into cDNA by an enzyme called reverse transcriptase in order to construct a cDNA library. Any cell or tissue can be used to construct a genomic library, since the whole genome exists in every somatic cell. However, mRNA is processed differently in each cell so that a cDNA library constructed from mRNA is different for each tissue or for each cell. An alveolar type 2 cell cDNA library contains only those genes expressed in type 2 cells and differs from a lung fibroblast cDNA library.

Restriction enzymes are the key to cutting DNA into pieces that can be inserted or ligated into vectors. The restriction enzyme cuts can be blunt-ended or staggered, but the DNA pieces are ligated most effectively into the

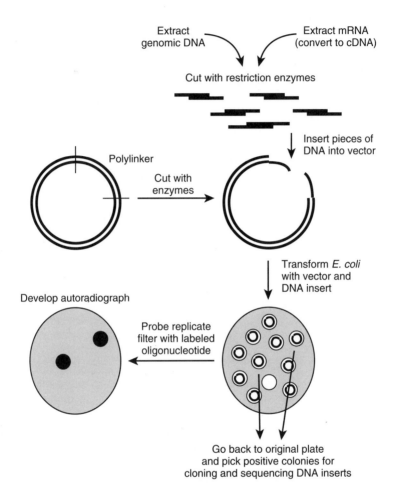

FIGURE 2–9. **Finding the INH Resistance Gene: Making a DNA Library.** Either genomic DNA or cDNA that has been reverse transcribed from mRNA is extracted and cut with restriction enzymes. Genomic DNA produces a genomic library containing DNA regulatory, as well as protein coding, information. The cDNA library contains no DNA regulatory information. The pieces of DNA are inserted into a vector (see Fig. 2–10) and the vector is transfected into bacteria such as *Escherichia coli*. Once the bacteria, each containing a single piece of transfected DNA, have grown to fill the plate, a replicate filter is made of the bacterial colonies, and the filter is probed with a radiolabeled oligonucleotide or cDNA that identifies by hybridization the DNA of interest. The colonies containing the DNA of interest are then identified on the plate of bacteria. They are lifted from the plate and cloned, producing many bacteria expressing only the DNA species of interest. Screening the library under high-stringency conditions reveals only DNA that is identical to that of the probe. Screening under low-stringency conditions reveals related DNA species.

vector if the ends are staggered and therefore cohesive or sticky. Since most vectors are constructed so that they contain multiple restriction sites, the circular vectors are opened by the same enzyme as was used to cut the DNA into pieces. This results in DNA strands that are complementary to those in the vector, allowing efficient hybridization between the two. The piece of DNA to be inserted into the vector is then pasted into the open vector site with a DNA ligase enzyme (Fig. 2–10).

Depending on the restriction enzyme used (rare versus frequent cutters), the fragments of DNA are either small for frequent cutters or large for rare cutters. Large fragments of DNA are more likely to contain whole genes, or at least the major portions of genes; frequent cutters are more likely to produce smaller pieces of genes. Plasmids can readily accept only small fragments of DNA, up to 1 kb, whereas bacterial phage vectors can accept DNA as large as 15 kb. Cosmids, which are hybrids of plasmids and phage vectors, can accept DNA fragments of 15 to 45 kb, and yeast artificial chromosome (YAC) vectors can accept huge pieces of DNA, up to 1000 kb. The latter are valuable in screening large pieces of chromosomal DNA when looking at gene linkage but are less useful in focusing on a single gene.

To produce a DNA library, bacteria *(E. coli)* are transfected (transformed) with the vectors containing fragments of DNA of different sizes; each vector contains only one DNA fragment but the vectors contain overlapping pieces of DNA that cover the whole genome, in this case the whole genome of INH-sensitive mycobacteria. Once the bacteria containing different fragments of DNA grow to nearly cover the culture plate, replicate filters are made by overlaying a piece of nylon or nitrocellulose on the plate. The DNA transferred to the filter is then denatured to convert it to single-stranded DNA and is immobilized on the filter and screened for the gene of interest with a radiolabeled cDNA probe that will hybridize to those bacterial colonies containing the piece of DNA recognized by the probe (Fig. 2–11). If this sounds like a Southern blot of each of the colonies on the filter paper, that is what it is. Those colonies, or plaques, containing the DNA of interest are then matched to colonies on the original plate and lifted from the plate;

DNA inserted into vector polylinker site with DNA ligase

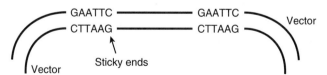

FIGURE 2–10. **Inserting DNA into a Vector.** Double-stranded DNA is inserted into a vector by cutting the vector open with an appropriate restriction enzyme (either chosen to match the ends of the inserted DNA or so that similar restriction sites are not present in the inserted DNA so that it is not cut into pieces). Sticky, overlapping ends of DNA and vector are preferred for ligation. A DNA ligase is added to seal the DNA into the vector site. As noted in Figure 2–8, many vectors now have polylinker sites that provide multiple restriction enzyme cutting sites.

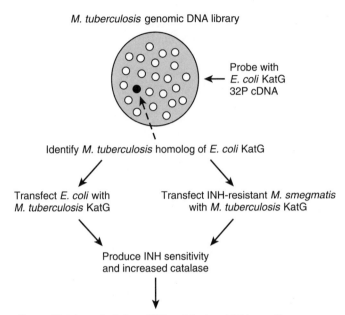

FIGURE 2–11. **Finding the INH Resistance Gene.** Once the DNA library of INH-sensitive *M. tuberculosis* is made, it is screened with a probe from the *E. coli KatG* gene at low stringency to identify the *M. tuberculosis KatG* homolog. The *M. tuberculosis KatG* cDNA is then transfected into INH-resistant *E. coli* and *M. smegmatis,* making each INH-sensitive and incidentally increasing their catalase activity. Lastly, *M. tuberculosis* isolates from a number of patients are screened for the presence of *KatG*; the INH-resistant isolates are found to have no *KatG*. The exact mutation in *KatG* cannot be identified, but a tool is now available to determine if INH resistance is the result of absent *KatG*.

these colonies are then grown so that the DNA in the positive bacterial colony can be isolated and sequenced. As discussed in Chapter 1, hybridization can be carried out at varying stringencies. High-stringency screening favors hybridization and identification of DNA with high sequence similarity to the probe. Low-stringency screening allows identification of pieces of DNA or genes that are similar but not identical to the DNA or gene represented by the probe. In crossing species, one may want to use a low- rather than high-stringency screen in order to pick up species-homologous genes.

It is unlikely that the complete gene is present in a single colony, especially if it is a large gene, so one may have to clone and sequence several colonies identified by the probe and then piece together the resulting DNA information to determine the structure of the complete gene. In some instances, pieces of the gene may not have been identified by the original probe, and one may need to repeat the screening of the library with a new probe to find all of the gene.

In the search for the INH resistance gene, the cDNA probes constructed from the *E. coli* peroxidase gene were used to screen a genomic library of INH-sensitive *M. tuberculosis* (see Fig. 2–11). One of the probes identified several colonies containing pieces of DNA that when transfected into INH-resistant, low–catalase producing organisms, converted them to INH-sensitive high-catalase producers. The DNA in these colonies was cloned and then sequenced. *Cloning* involves growing many bacteria from a single bacterium transfected with a unique piece of a gene to form a large colony of bacteria all containing the same unique piece of DNA. Sequencing the cloned DNA that induced INH sensitivity revealed that the DNA was similar to the *E. coli* hydroperoxidase gene *(katG)*. Mutations in *M. tuberculosis katG* that abolished catalase activity also altered the ability of the gene to confer INH sensitivity to resistant organisms. Lastly, the *M. tuberculosis katG* probe was used on a Northern blot of RNA extracted from a number of clinical isolates of INH-sensitive and -resistant organisms. All of the INH-sensitive organisms expressed *M. tuberculosis katG* mRNA, but there was complete loss of *katG* mRNA in the INH-resistant organisms. Thus, in these patients some form of mutation that resulted in deletion of *katG* may have led to INH resistance. The presumed role of *katG* is to produce catalase, which is thought to be important in converting INH to its metabolically active form.

A number of recent studies have used molecular techniques to define the major mutations in the *M. tuberculosis* genome that leads to resistance to rifampin, streptomycin, and pyrazinamide. Rifampin interferes with transcription of mycobacterial RNA by binding to the β subunit of RNA polymerase. Mutations in *M. tuberculosis* RNA polymerase (encoded by the *rpoB* gene) account for greater than 95% of rifampicin-resistant cases of *M. tuberculosis*. Mutations in the *M. tuberculosis rpsL* gene, which encodes a ribosomal protein, and in the *rrs* gene, which encodes 16s rRNA, account for two thirds of streptomycin resistance. Pyrazinamide, which acts primarily on dormant rather than actively multiplying mycobacteria, requires a bacterial amidase to convert it to its active form. The amidase is encoded by the *pncA* gene. The amidase is inactive in pyrazinamide-resistant TB, and the gene is mutated in these bacteria.

## Determining the Mutations in Resistant *Mycobacterium tuberculosis*

Since many of the mutations in *M. tuberculosis* genes that lead to drug resistance have been described recently, there are as yet few studies of the frequency of these mutations in large samples of single-drug and multidrug-resistant mycobacteria. One recent international study of multidrug-resistant samples found that of 44 streptomycin-resistant strains, 25 had *rpsL* mutations and 5 had *rrs* mutations. Thus one third were resistant on the basis of as yet undescribed mutations. In contrast, 28 of the 29 rifampin-resistant organisms had *rpoB* mutations. Of the 42 INH-resistant strains, 20 had *katG* mutations and 5 had *inhA* mutations; thus, 40% had yet to be described mutations responsible for INH resistance. Eighty-five per cent of the multi-drug-resistant isolates had several mutations, suggesting that the primary mechanism responsible for multidrug resistance is an accumulation of mutations in specific genes that are the target of drugs, rather than the appearance of a novel mutation that affects transport or metabolism of all drugs.

The approach to determining specific mutations that was used in these studies provides an opportunity to discuss a highly sensitive technique for

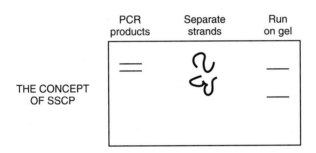

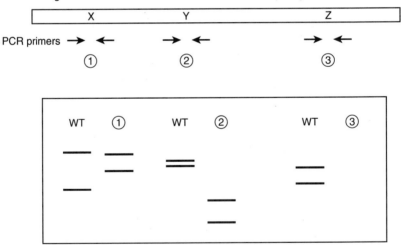

FIGURE 2–12. **SSCP and Drug Resistance.** PCR products run on a typical denaturing gel are shown on the left. For SSCP, PCR products are separated by heat and allowed to renature, reconforming and assuming a shape that is dictated by the charge interaction of individual bases. The migration of the DNA strands in a nondenaturing gel (on the right) is a function of both the size of DNA fragments and the shape of the reconformed DNA fragments. One can use PCR primers that will amplify previously determined sites of DNA mutations conferring resistance to INH or rifampin (X,Y,Z). Wild-type (drug-sensitive) mycobacteria are run as controls. A single base pair substitution or deletion can lead to a change in conformation of the renatured products and a different pattern of migration in the gel. In example 3 a mutation at the primer sites results in lack of a PCR product.

diagnosing gene mutations. The luciferase assay discussed previously has the potential to define the antibiotics to which an organism is resistant. By using PCR-based methods, one can amplify and sequence pieces of DNA from genes known to be mutated in INH or rifampin resistance. Although this approach is time-consuming, the increasing availability of automated DNA sequencing makes it feasible. However, the preceding study used single strand conformational polymorphism (SSCP) to determine which genes were mutated in each *M. tuberculosis* isolate (Fig. 2–12). This method uses PCR to amplify a known portion of a gene, whose mutation is suspected; for example, the 27 codons of the *rpoB* gene known to be responsible for rifampin resistance. The resulting double strands of amplified DNA are then separated into single strands by heat. The single strands undergo conformational changes determined by the sequence of bases in the DNA, in a manner similar to that occurring when bases on opposite DNA strands interact with one another (A to T, C to G). This base binding creates secondary and tertiary structures that determine, along with size, how a piece of DNA will migrate under nondenaturing conditions. Mutations in a single base can alter the way in which single-stranded DNA conforms and subsequently migrates in a gel. If no mutation has occurred, the area of *rpoB* that is amplified in DNA from a resistant organism will be the same as that of a sensitive organism, and the DNA single strands migrate similarly. If a single base is altered, the DNA strand of the resistant organism migrates either faster or slower than that of the sensitive organism. The method does not provide information about what mutation has occurred, only that there is a mutation in the amplified portion of the *rpoB* gene. Direct sequencing would be necessary to determine the actual mutation that has occurred. Although there have been a large number of mutations described in *rpoB*, they all occur within a limited area of *rpoB*, and missense mutations in codons for two amino acids 12 bases apart account for 80% of reported instances of rifampin resistance.

## SUGGESTED READING

### Polymerase Chain Reaction and Diagnosis of *Mycobacterium Tuberculosis* Infection

Richeldi L, Barnini S, Saltini C: Molecular diagnosis of tuberculosis. Eur Respir J Suppl 8:689s–700s, 1995.

Roth A, Schaberg T, Mauch H: Molecular diagnosis of tuberculosis: Current clinical validity and future perspectives. Eur Respir J 10:1877–1891, 1997.

Schluger NW, Rom WN: The polymerase chain reaction in the diagnosis and evaluation of pulmonary infections. Am J Respir Crit Care Med 152:11–16, 1995.

### Epidemiology and DNA Fingerprinting

Alland D, Kalkut GE, Moss AR, et al: Transmission of tuberculosis in New York City. An analysis by DNA fingerprinting and conventional methods. N Engl J Med 330:1710–1716, 1994.

Small PM, Hopewell PC, Singh SP, et al: The epidemiology of tuberculosis in San Francisco. A population-based study using conventional and molecular methods. N Engl J Med 330:1703–1709, 1994.

van Sooligen D, Hermans PWM: Epidemiology of tuberculosis by DNA fingerprinting. Eur Respir J Suppl 8:649s–656s, 1995.

**Reporter Genes and Luciferase**

Jacobs WR, Barletta RG, Udani R, et al: Rapid assessment of drug susceptibilities of *Mycobacterium tuberculosis* by means of luciferase reporter phages. [accompanying editorial] Science 260:819–822, 1993.

**Mechanisms of Drug Resistance**

Banerjee A, Dubnau E, Quemard A, et al: *InhA*, a gene encoding a target for isoniazid and ethionamide in *Mycobacterium tuberculosis*. Science 264:227–230, 1994.

Cole ST, Telenti A: Drug resistance in *Mycobacterium tuberculosis*. Eur Respir J Suppl 8:701s–713, 1995.

Donnabella V, Martiniuk F, Kinney D, et al: Isolation of the gene for the β subunit of RNA polymerase from rifampicin-resistant *Mycobacterium tuberculosis* and identification of new mutations. Am J Respir Cell Mol Biol 11:639–643, 1994.

Morris S, Han Bai G, Suffys P, et al: Molecular mechanisms of multiple drug resistance in clinical isolates of *Mycobacterium tuberculosis*. J Infect Dis 171:954–960, 1995.

Sninnick TM, King CH, Quinn FD: Molecular biology, virulence and pathogenicity of mycobacteria. Am J Med Sci 309:92–98, 1995.

Zhang Y, Heym B, Allen B, et al: The catalase-peroxidase gene and isoniazid resistance of *Mycobacterium tuberculosis*. Nature 358:591–593, 1992.

# Neuromuscular Diseases: Amyotrophic Lateral Sclerosis

chromosomes • linkage analysis • recombination • genetic markers • DNA sequencing • transgenic mice • site-directed mutagenesis • gain of function mutations • apoptosis

Anyone who has spent time in an intensive care unit or has dealt with patients in respiratory failure has been involved with, at some point, the agonizing decision of whether to institute ventilatory support in a patient with some form of hereditary muscle disease that has affected respiratory muscles, leading to life-threatening hypoxia or hypercapnia. Many of these patients are young and will require ventilatory support for the rest of their lives. Often, other family members have suffered similar fates.

Muscular dystrophies and amyotrophic lateral sclerosis (ALS) are two of the most frequent forms of hereditary muscle disease leading to respiratory failure. In each, a considerable amount of information has been generated by molecular biologic techniques over the past few years. Some of the methods used to generate this new information are discussed in this chapter.

ALS is the motor neuron disease responsible for Lou Gehrig's premature retirement from baseball. It usually begins with asymmetric lower extremity weakness and progresses to complete paralysis within 5 years. Paralysis is due to degeneration of large motor neurons of the brain and spinal cord. Ten per cent of the cases are familial autosomal dominant disease (familial ALS or FALS), which resembles in every way the sporadic form of ALS. Recent studies have identified a mutation in the Cu/Zn superoxide dismutase gene that is associated with some, but not all, cases of FALS. This observation provides a clue as to the cause of at least some cases of ALS and also provides an opportunity to discuss in this chapter important molecular biologic concepts such as chromosome structure, linkage analysis, genetic markers, transgenic animals, DNA sequencing, and site-directed mutagenesis.

## Finding the Superoxide Dismutase Gene: Linkage Analysis

Humans have a total of 23 pairs of chromosomes, including the X and Y sex chromosomes. The 50,000 to 100,000 genes making up the $3 \times 10^9$ base pairs of the human genome are tightly packed into these 23 chromosomes. One chromosome of the pair is inherited from each parent. Each chromosome, viewed best at mitosis, has a constricted region (the centromere) that holds the sister pairs of chromatids together and creates a long arm and a short arm on each chromosome. The chromosomes contain areas of nucleotides rich in A-T and G-C that stain differently with specific dyes to produce a characteristic banding pattern for each chromosome (Fig. 3–1). These and other staining bands (some high-resolution methods reveal as many as 800 bands per chromosome) and the division into long and short arms provide a nomenclature for depicting the chromosomal locations of genes. For example, the location of one gene identified as being important in FALS is 21q22.1: q stands for the long arm (versus p for the short arm) of chromosome 21; 2 stands for the second region of chromosome 21; 2 stands for the second bands in region 2; and .1 stands for the first subset within that band. As can be seen in Figure 3–1, chromosomes are of different length; chromosome 1 accounts for 8% of the human genome, whereas the Y chromosome accounts for 2%.

How does one go about finding the chromosome on which a gene associated with a specific disease or biologic process is located? If the gene has been cloned, one can perform in situ hybridization with a labeled cRNA probe on a slide of mitotic chromosomes (see Chapter 8) to locate the gene of interest to a general area of the chromosome.

If one does not know the identity of the gene—for example, the gene that causes ALS—the method of choice for identifying it is linkage analysis, and the key is the map of the human genome. (Chapter 10 discusses the human genome project and Chapter 6 addresses positional cloning and chro-

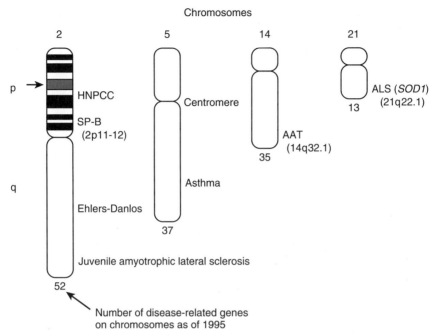

FIGURE 3–1. **Map of Human Chromosomes.** Schematic presentation of four chromosomes with pulmonary disease–related genes. (See also Figs. 6–2 and 7–16 for chromosomes 7 and 3, respectively.) Only one pair of the two chromosomal partners is shown. Chromosomes are depicted according to relative size; actually they are numbered by size, with 1 being the largest and 22 being the smallest. Chromosomal G (Giemsa) bands are actually varying shades of gray representing varying concentrations of AT nucleotides. Only the 2p banding pattern is shown. These bands contain from 5000 to 10,000,000 nucleotides. The X chromosome, which is about three times the size of the Y chromosome, contains some 150 million bases and 2000 to 5000 genes. Genes tend to be in the 5000- to 25,000-nucleotide range, although the largest known gene, the Duchenne's muscular dystrophy gene, is 2.5 million base pairs. HNPCC, hereditary nonpolyposis colon carcinoma.

mosome jumping and walking, which is the process of moving along a chromosome to discover a disease-causing gene.) ALS provides a perfect opportunity to discuss the concept of linkage analysis.

The search for a cause of ALS was made easier by the presence of "junk" DNA, which in the human consists in part of simple repeating sequences of nucleotides that appear at various intervals throughout the genome and serve little apparent function. Some repeats appear as genes, for example, the $\alpha$-globulin gene appears twice and ribosomal RNA (rRNA) appears many times and is located on several chromosomes. However, most repeats occur within junk DNA. There is a large ALU sequence of approximately 300 base pairs (cut by the restriction enzyme alu) that appears thousands of times in the genome. Most repeats are more simple, however, consisting of two to five base pairs. These are called simple tandem repeats, the most frequent being an AC *dinucleotide repeat* that appears at various intervals 50,000 to 100,000 times in the genome. A genetic map of more than 3000 of these *microsatellite markers* has been assembled, and it can be used for linkage analysis of genes that may lie close to these markers (see Fig. 7–16 for other uses of these microsatellite sequences).

Mendel stated that an individual's genes are inherited independently of one another by their offspring. This is true unless the genes are located on the same chromosome in proximity to one another. In this case, genes tend to be inherited together; the closer two genes or pieces of DNA are on the chromosome, the more likely they are to be coinherited. Since the dinucleotide repeats noted earlier are so common throughout the genome, almost any gene has a number of markers close by. The relation of such a marker to a defective gene can be used to trace inheritance of the gene through families and generate data for linkage analysis.

*Crossing over* is key to providing markers for linkage analysis. During the meiotic phase of cell division, the two chromosomes come together, make contact at specific points, and exchange homologous segments. This involves crossing over of the two chromosomes and homologous recombination of parts of each chromosome (Fig. 3–2). This exchange of chromosomal material during meiotic cell division is responsible for much of the genetic diversity in humans (see Fig. 4–1 for more detail on meiotic recombination). It can also be used as a tool for finding genes. The farther apart two genetic elements are, the more likely they are to separate from one another during crossover and recombination. Alternatively, the closer two genetic elements are, the more likely they are to cosegregate, that is, stay together. If a gene and a marker—for example a particular dinucleotide repeat—are coinherited more than 50% of the time, they are likely genetically linked and on the same chromosome. If they are coinherited more than 99% of the time, they are not only on the same chromosome but also are by definition within 1 centimorgan (cM) of one another. A *centimorgan* is a chromosomal map unit but is on average 1000 kb or $10^6$ base pairs. By following the frequency of coinherited loci in families, one can determine statistically how far apart the two loci are on the chromosome. Linkage analysis now uses computer programs analyzing large pedigrees over several generations for the likelihood of occurrence of a disease phenotype in association with a polymorphic marker. Likelihood of linkage is expressed as a logarithm of the odds (LOD) score, which if greater than 3 favors linkage over chance by a factor of 1000.

Using this approach to follow the linkage between the occurrence of FALS and dinucleotide markers in FALS families, investigators recently found that a subset of individuals with FALS mapped with a dinucleotide repeat on chromosome 21q22.1, in an area close to the gene coding for the cytosolic antioxidant enzyme Cu/Zn superoxide dismutase *(SOD1)*. There is considerable indirect evidence that a defect in *SOD1* might be involved in ALS. Some ALS patients have lower than normal levels of *SOD1* in their red blood cells and cerebrospinal fluid, and there is evidence that free radicals can induce

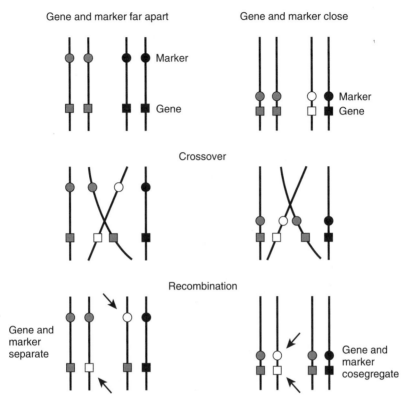

FIGURE 3–2. **Chromosomal Crossover and Recombination.** During meiosis, chromosomes actually touch and exchange pieces of DNA. As many as three such events occur on each chromosome per meiotic cell division. This process provides a way of following linkage between a disease and a marker gene. In this figure, the boxes represent the gene of interest, with the open box being the mutant, disease-causing gene. The circles represent a marker, in this instance a dinucleotide repeat of a certain length. If the mutant gene is transferred from one chromosome to another and the marker repeat is far from the gene, as in the diagram on the left, the two will not track together *(arrows)*. Thus, one person will acquire the disease carried by the open gene but will not express the marker. In the example on the right, the disease-carrying mutant gene and marker are close together, so persons who inherit the disease will also carry the marker gene *(arrows)*. The more often persons with the disease also carry the marker gene, the closer the marker gene is to the disease-causing gene.

neurodegeneration and neuronal cell death in vitro. Once the possibility of FALS linkage to *SOD1* was considered, investigators cloned and sequenced portions of the *SOD1* gene and reported mutations in four of the five *SOD1* exons, although none of the mutations was in the active site of the enzyme and none was a null mutation, that is, mutations that stopped production of the SOD1 protein (see further on for a discussion of DNA mutations). The 20 mutations in *SOD1* that have been reported to date are so-called missense mutations, causing a change in a single amino acid. *SOD* enzyme activity is usually in the 25 to 50% of normal range in these individuals. There are no mutations in *SOD1*, and *SOD1* activity is normal in control individuals and in FALS families in whom there is no linkage to chromosome 21q.

Since cytosolic Cu/Zn superoxide dismutase is an important antioxidant enzyme that detoxifies or causes dismutation of superoxide anion to hydrogen peroxide, which is itself then detoxified (Fig. 3–3), investigators were encouraged that at least some FALS patients, and perhaps some patients with sporadic cases of ALS, had motor neuron degeneration that resulted from oxidant damage and that treatment of ALS patients with antioxidants might be at hand. Indeed, it was felt that mutations in other Cu/Zn superoxide dismutase enzymes such as mitochondrial manganese-dependent superoxide dismutase and extracellular Cu/Zn superoxide dismutase might account for the remaining cases of FALS and sporadic ALS.

## Mutations: Types and Consequences

Mutations in DNA are of two major types: point mutations and insertion-deletion mutations. *Point mutations* involve a simple change of one nucleotide for another. A change in a single nucleotide may have no effect on the protein produced; a change in the third nucleotide of a codon GUU to GUC or GUA or GUG has no effect on the amino acid produced because all these triplets code for valine (see Fig. 1–8). In contrast, some point mutations can profoundly alter translation of the code into protein and the formation of RNA

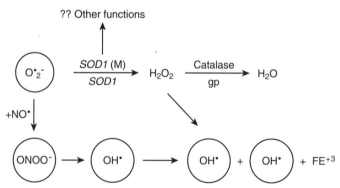

FIGURE 3–3. **Function of Normal and Mutant *SOD1*.** Superoxide anion ($O_2^-$) undergoes dismutation by *SOD1* to $H_2O_2$, which, in turn, becomes $H_2O$ in the presence of catalase. Circles identify toxic radicals. The mutations in *SOD1* that are associated with familial amyotrophic lateral sclerosis (FALS) lead to small changes in Cu/Zn superoxide dismutase activity but do not appear to cause disease because of decreased dismutase activity. Rather, some other function of the mutant *SOD1* appears to lead to motor neuron death; thus the term gain of function mutation.

itself. Figure 3–4 shows that a single point mutation can lead to a *nonsense mutation*, that is, can introduce a premature stop codon that terminates translation; produce a simple change in amino acids; or alter the RNA splicing mechanisms (see Fig. 6–5 for further illustration of RNA splicing), thereby changing the post-transcriptional processing of RNA, potentially producing entirely different proteins. *Insertion-deletion* mutations involve the elimination or addition of one or more nucleotides, which can have the effect of deleting an amino acid codon or *shifting the reading frame* so that the whole translation process is altered.

## DNA Sequencing: Finding and Identifying Mutations

This is a good place to discuss how one detects and defines DNA mutations in the first place. (See Chapter 6 for further definition of the types of DNA mutations and Chapter 7 for further discussion on the detection of mutations.) This chapter presents the technique of DNA sequencing, which is used to define the specific mutations involved in various diseases. DNA sequencing is also crucial in determining DNA structure as well as to virtually every aspect of DNA technology. There is certainly plenty of DNA to sequence, since the human genome consists of $10^9$ base pairs. Increasingly, automated sequencing has been substituted for the rather laborious methods that were in use only a few years ago. The principles are similar and are illustrated in Figure 3–5. In both types of sequencing, the ingredients consist of *a single-stranded DNA template* to which *a primer* has been annealed, *DNA polymerase,* and *dideoxynucleotide precursors* for all four DNA bases. Dideoxynucleotides lack the 3′ OH group that is required for DNA chain elongation. Thus, when the dideoxynucleotide is incorporated, DNA synthesis is terminated at that point. In practice, the DNA fragment to be sequenced is cloned into a vector and the mixture is heated to cause strands to separate. A radiolabeled primer is then annealed to the DNA fragment, preventing it from reinserting into the vector as double-stranded DNA. The DNA-primer mixture is separated into four tubes to which a DNA polymerase and *all four deoxynucleotide triphosphates* (adenosine triphosphate, thymidine triphosphate, cytidine triphosphate, and guanine triphosphate) are added. DNA polymerase is added to each tube, and each tube receives a different dideoxynucleotide, which when incorporated into the growing DNA chain terminates DNA synthesis because the dideoxynucleotide does not present a hydroxyl group at its 3′ end for attachment of subsequent nucleotides. Since the dideoxynucleotide terminates the reaction, the specific dideoxynucleotide added determines the last nucleotide added to the 3′ end of the chain. The polymerase directs copy of the DNA template in a complementary fashion, starting at the 5′ primer and moving in a 3′ direction until a dideoxynucleotide is added, terminating the reaction. Since a different dideoxynucleotide is added to each tube, the

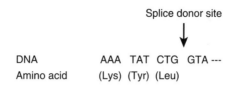

Point mutations

Splice donor site

DNA       AAA  TAT  CTG  GTA ---
Amino acid    (Lys) (Tyr) (Leu)

| Nonsense | Missense | RNA splicing |
|---|---|---|
| AAA  TA(A)  CTG | AAA  (G)AT  CTG | AAA  TAT  CTG  (C)TA  AGG |
| (Lys) ((Stop)) | (Lys) ((Asp)) (Leu) | (Lys) (Tyr) (Leu) ((Leu))((Arg)) |

Insertion-deletion Mutations

DNA       AAA  TAT  GTG  ATT  CCC
Amino acid    (Lys) (Try) (Val) (Ile) (Pro)

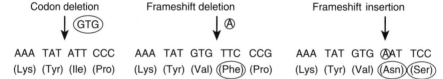

| Codon deletion | Frameshift deletion | Frameshift insertion |
|---|---|---|
| ↓ (GTG) | ↓ (A) | ↓ |
| AAA  TAT  ATT  CCC | AAA  TAT  GTG  TTC  CCG | AAA  TAT  GTG  (A)AT  TCC |
| (Lys) (Tyr) (Ile) (Pro) | (Lys) (Tyr) (Val) ((Phe)) (Pro) | (Lys) (Tyr) (Val) ((Asn))((Ser)) |

FIGURE 3–4. **Major Types of DNA Mutations.** There are two major types of DNA mutations: point and insertion/deletion mutations. The top line represents DNA triplet codons for the amino acids in parentheses. The arrow indicates a GTA donor splice site (see Chapter 6 for discussion of splicing). In each example of point mutations, there is a single substitution of one nucleotide for another. As discussed in the text, some mutations (especially in the third position) will produce no change in the coded amino acid. In the example of nonsense mutations, substitution of an A (circled) for a T in the second triplet produces a stop codon that terminates translation of the message and therefore truncates the protein. In the missense mutation, a G (circled) substituted for the first T of the second codon changes one amino acid (tyrosine) into another (asparagine). In the RNA splicing example, substitution of a C (circled) for the G at the splice donor site eliminates the splice site and creates a new protein with additional amino acids (leucine, arginine, and so on). Insertion/deletion mutations are illustrated in the lower half of the figure. Codon deletions eliminate a triplet codon and therefore an amino acid in protein. Frameshift deletions eliminate a nucleotide, in this case the A (circled) of the fourth triplet codon, changing the ATT codon to a TTC and an isoleucine to a phenylalanine, as the C from the fifth codon becomes part of the fourth codon. The fifth codon also changes, as a G from the normal sixth codon (not shown) becomes part of the fifth codon. In this example, the change of CCC to CCG does not alter the amino acid because both code for proline. In the frameshift insertion example, a single nucleotide A (circled) is inserted at the first position of the fourth codon to change the ATT (isoleucine) to an AAT (asparagine), pushing the T to a new TCC codon that results in a serine instead of a proline.

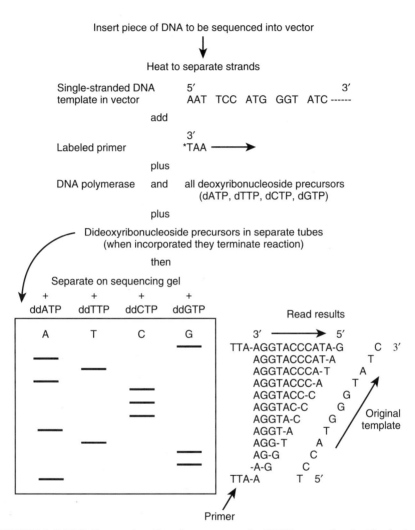

FIGURE 3–5. **DNA Sequencing.** Complementary strands of DNA are produced with selective nucleotides that do not support elongation. In each of four tubes, a labeled primer (reading from 3′ to 5′) is annealed to the single-stranded (SS) DNA template. DNA polymerase in the presence of all four nucleosides initiates copying of the template. A different *di*deoxynucleoside is added to each tube, which when incorporated into the elongating DNA chain terminates the reaction at that specific nucleoside. The labeled chains of DNA in each tube are separated on an agarose gel and the synthesized chains migrate according to their length. Each chain in the ddATP tube ends with an A, each chain in the ddTTP tube ends with a T, and so on. The sequence of the copied template can then be read from bottom to top of the gel as shown. The original DNA is complementary to the synthesized DNA (see text for further explanation).

length of the growing chain is different in each tube. The newly synthesized DNA from each tube is then denatured and each is separated by electrophoresis in a gel. The sequence of the synthesized complementary strand can be read directly from the autoradiograph using the radiolabeled primer as the marker. The shortest strand of DNA, the strands closest to the 5' primer, runs the fastest in the gel, so the gel is read 5' to 3' from the bottom up. Because of limitations in the size of gels, one can usually sequence only 500 bases at a time.

Automated sequencing procedures are rapidly replacing the preceding method, which is labor-intensive, especially when one sequences both DNA strands. The automated procedure is similar in principle, except that the dideoxynucleotides are each labeled by a different fluorescent tag, each of which carries a spectrally distinct fluor. All of the four reaction mixtures can be run in the same tube, since each dideoxynucleotide produces a different color. The strands are separated in a sequencing gel and passed through a laser that excites, and a photomultiplier tube that reads, fluorescence. All the information is then processed in a computer that translates the color information from the gel into a nucleic acid sequence. This method is now in common use for small projects, such as determining the site or type of mutation in a gene of interest, but is also being applied to sequencing large segments of DNA in various genome projects.

## Making Mutations: The Key to Understanding Gene Function

One can now produce or engineer genes with any mutation desired. This ability to target a change in DNA nucleic acid sequence, and thus in mRNA-directed protein synthesis, relies on a technique called site-directed mutagenesis. This technique is one of the most frequently used molecular tools. It allows one to define in detail mechanisms of gene regulation and gene and protein function, to add or subtract restriction sites in DNA, and to create the transgenes used in the ALS experiments discussed earlier. Mutants can be created that will add stop codons to DNA, and therefore mRNA, by introducing a premature ATC that will stop translation of a protein. Single nucleotide mutations can be introduced to examine the specificity of transcription factor binding sites in the regulation of DNA transcription (see Chapter 8) or of regulation of protein structure such as in the case of the cystic fibrosis transport regulator (see Chapter 6). In the instance of ALS transgenic mice, a human *SOD1* DNA was engineered that introduced an ALA to VAL substitution at the 4 position of *SOD1* or a GLY to ALA substitution at the 93rd amino acid of *SOD1*. These are the most frequent *SOD1* mutations found in FALS patients.

Random mutagenesis can be induced in genes by damaging DNA with chemicals or radiation, but this does not allow one to mutagenize a specific gene or region of a gene. Although there are now a number of ways to produce site-directed mutagenesis, the most commonly used approach is to create a synthetic oligonucleotide with one or more nucleotides that differ from the normal (wild-type) DNA or with a whole new sequence that has been added or eliminated. The oligonucleotides can be created by a programmable nucleic acid synthesizing machine that makes chains up to 100 nucleotides in length. The method, illustrated in Figure 3–6, involves fitting the synthesized oligonucleotide into a plasmid vector and then infecting *Escherichia coli* with the vector in order to grow large amounts of the mutagenized

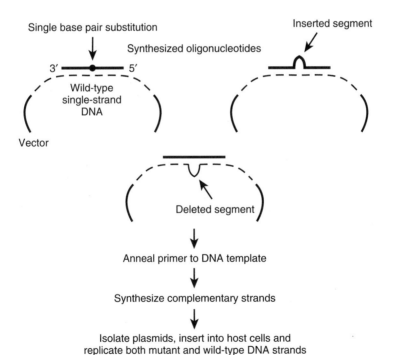

FIGURE 3–6. **Making DNA Mutations.** Oligonucleotides with various types of mutation (thick line) are synthesized and annealed to the original DNA, which is in a vector. The oligonucleotide is incorporated into a newly synthesized strand and then grown in bacteria, identified, and isolated for use (see text for further explanation).

DNA for use. The trick, and molecular biology always involves clever technical tricks, is to separate the double-stranded vector DNA by heat and to anneal the single-stranded mutant oligonucleotide into the vector under low-stringency conditions that allow binding of similar but not exactly complementary nucleic acids. New strands of DNA that incorporate the mutant oligonucleotide are then synthesized with the help of a DNA polymerase. The vectors containing the inserted material are then grown in bacteria, with the bacterial colonies containing the new DNA being identified. The mutated DNA can be extracted from the bacteria and is then available for microinjection and production of transgenic animals or for study in transfected cells.

## Transgenic Mice Prove *SOD1* Mutation Represents Gain of Function

There are several parts of the theory that decreased Cu/Zn superoxide dismutase activity causes ALS that did not quite fit. Most importantly, mutations that lead to loss of protein function are usually inherited in a recessive fashion, that is, both genes on a chromosome (both alleles) must be abnormal, since the presence of one normal allele would produce sufficient enzyme activity to maintain normal function. FALS is inherited in a dominant fashion, and therefore gain of function (appearance of a new function), perhaps from an abnormal protein product produced by the mutant gene, rather than loss of function might be expected.

It was experiments using transgenic mice that provided a whole new direction for research in ALS. The trick in these experiments was to produce transgenic mice that expressed either normal or mutant human *SOD1* without interfering with the production of normal mouse sod1. The transgenic mice turned out to have normal mouse sod protein. However, those with the mutant human gene, but not the normal human gene, acquired classic ALS, which was first manifested as hind limb weakness at 3 to 4 months of age; the mice then became paralyzed and died within a month. The pathologic muscle features were similar to those in human ALS. In fact, those mice with the largest amount of mutant human protein had the most virulent and rapidly progressive muscle disease. It is unclear how the mutant forms of *SOD1* induce neuronal degeneration, but most investigators believe that the mutant proteins may result in increased generation of free radicals from $H_2O_2$ or may facilitate formation of other toxic substances such as peroxynitrite involving the nitric oxide system (see Fig. 3–3). The results of a number of these experiments clearly support the gain of function disease hypothesis.

The transgenic mouse model of ALS not only focuses on a possible mechanism of disease but also provides an animal model for testing various forms of therapy.

How does one go about making a *transgenic mouse* (Fig. 3–7), a mouse into which foreign genes have been introduced? *Transgenes* are linear strands

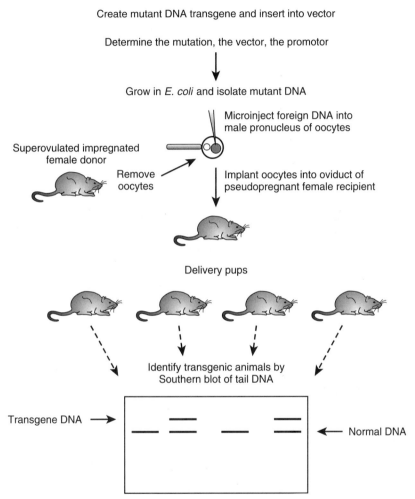

FIGURE 3–7. **Making a Transgenic Mouse.** A mutation of interest is created in DNA and the mutant DNA is ligated (as illustrated in Fig. 3–6) into an appropriate vector. In creating the transgene, one must consider the mutation to be produced, the vector to use (see Fig. 2–8), and whether the transgene is to be expressed in all cells using a universal promoter or is to be expressed in only certain cells by using a cell-specific promoter. The vector infects *Escherichia coli*, where large amounts of DNA are grown and purified. This DNA is then placed into the male pronucleus of oocytes taken from a superovulated impregnated female mouse by microinjection, and the oocytes carrying the transgene are placed into the oviduct of a female mouse that has mated with a sterile male. The pups that are produced are then typed by analysis of tail DNA on a Southern blot using a probe that recognizes the normal and the mutant DNA. Heterozygotes can then be mated to produce homozygotes.

of DNA that when introduced into cells are integrated into the host chromosomes. If the modified chromosome is present in germ line cells (egg or sperm), the transgenes will be passed on to offspring of the mouse. In general, if foreign species transgenes are expressed, they will display only gain of function abnormalities, since the normal mouse gene will still be expressed. To produce loss of function, mice gene "knockout" methods have been developed and are discussed in Chapter 4.

Transgenic mice are produced by microinjecting several hundred copies of the mutated gene into the pronuclei of fertilized eggs that have been washed from the uterus of an impregnated female mouse. The injected eggs are transferred into the uterus of a pseudopregnant mouse—a mouse mated with a sterile male and primed with hormones to accept and implant the transferred eggs. The DNA integrates in a random fashion, usually in a tandem fashion (i.e., several repeats of the gene) at a single locus on a chromosome. For most experiments, the transgene has been engineered to contain the cDNA with the mutation of interest. If the transgene contains the normal regulatory information that guides time and place of expression, it is usually expressed in the cells that express the normal gene. The transgene can also be driven by a strong universal promoter and is then expressed in all tissues and cells, or it can be driven by a different cell-specific promoter, resulting in expression of the gene in a cell that does not normally express the gene. For example, using the SPC regulatory region will result in a gene being expressed in type 2 cells even if that gene is not normally expressed in type 2 cells. Animals that carry and express the transgene can be identified by a marker linked to the gene so that the cells that express the gene can be identified. Transgenic animals can by typed by extracting DNA from a tissue, usually a piece of the tail, and performing a Southern blot to prove that the DNA of interest is truly expressed in somatic cells of the animal. The mice can then be bred to produce homozygous or heterozygous transgenic mice.

The ALS transgenic mice carried the human *SOD1* driven by the SOD1 promoter. In one set of mice, one of two common *SOD1* mutations was introduced into the human gene. Transgenic mice expressing the normal human *SOD1* served as controls. Both forms of mutated *SOD1* genes resulted in an ALS-like disease, but the normal human *SOD1* caused no recognizable disease. In none of the animals was normal mouse SOD1 altered. The conclusion from these experiments was that mutated *SOD1* causes a gain of function disease. How mutant *SOD1* causes motor neuron damage and why these neurons are unique targets of this defective protein remain unclear at present, as do questions of whether mutations in other superoxide dismutase proteins account for any of the remaining FALS and sporadic ALS cases.

Transgenic animals have been used to explore the effects of gene mutations, as in this case; the effects of gene over expression; mechanisms of gene regulation; and functions of proteins. They have also been used as a means of producing foreign proteins for research and commercial purposes.

## *SOD1* Mutations Induce Programmed Cell Death: Apoptosis

A recent study using concepts and methods that we have already discussed has provided further data to show that mutant *SOD1* is functional and that the *SOD1* mutation is a gain of function mutation. This study also suggested a mechanism by which the mutant protein causes motor neuron disease.

It is clear from the discussions in Chapter 2 on tuberculosis that important genes are conserved across species. The *E. coli katG* gene was used to find a comparable *Mycobacterium tuberculosis* catalase gene that was important in the activation of isoniazid. Basic biologic processes such as cell division and development are regulated in a similar fashion in lower organisms and in humans (see Chapter 7 for discussion of studies in yeast that provided insights into cell cycle control in humans). The same conservation exists in protection against oxidant injury. A mutant form of yeast has been found that lacks Cu/Zn superoxide dismutase and is susceptible to oxidant damage. When this yeast is transfected with normal *SOD1*, the activity of the enzyme increases and the yeast is protected against oxidant injury. However, the same thing occurs when the yeast is transfected with either of two mutant forms of *SOD1*. Thus, mutant *SOD1* is functional in protecting against oxidant-induced injury, at least in yeast.

The next step was to overexpress mutant *SOD1* in a neuronal cell line. When these cells are maintained in the absence of serum, they die, and death occurs by a recently described mechanism called apoptosis, or programmed cell death. Overexpression of normal *wild-type SOD1*, achieved by transfecting the cells with *SOD1* driven by a strong constitutive promotor, prevented this cell death, suggesting that some change in the redox state of the cell associated with lack of serum induces apoptosis. When cells are transfected in a similar fashion with mutant *SOD1*, Cu/Zn superoxide dismutase activity rises as with normal *SOD1*, but the cells die at a much faster rate when serum is withdrawn. These observations (Fig. 3–8) suggest that apoptosis is mediated by reactive oxygen species and that the mutant *SOD1* was actually an inducer of apoptosis, likely via increased production of reactive oxygen species (see Fig. 3–3). Although the mechanism by which mutant *SOD1* might generate additional toxic radicals has not been worked out, neuronal cell death is the basis of ALS, and the mutant *SOD1* seems to play an important role in this process.

What is *apoptosis* and why has its discovery produced so much scientific interest? Until recently, a dying cell was just a dying cell—something bad happens to a cell, it loses the ability to control its volume and therefore swells, bursts, and dies, leaving behind cellular debris that generates an inflammatory reaction leading to phagocytosis. Once again information from a nonvertebrate system, along with studies of mammalian systems, has led to a totally new concept about cell death; programmed cell death or "death from within." This type of cell death, called apoptosis after the Greek word meaning

Mutant *SOD1* has antioxidant function

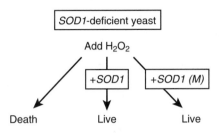

Mutant *SOD1* fosters apoptosis

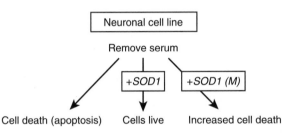

FIGURE 3–8. **The FALS *SOD1* Mutation Produces an Increased Cell Death Gain of Function.** Mutant *SOD1* (*SOD1 [M]*) in FALS patients has Cu/Zn superoxide dismutase activity, as demonstrated in yeast in this example. It appears to gain a cell-destructive function in that it fosters rather than prevents apoptosis of neuronal cells when serum is removed.

falling off, as leaves falling off of a tree, represents a morphologically and biochemically different form of cell death (Fig. 3–9). With apoptosis, cells shrink rather than swell, nuclear and cytoplasmic contents condense and fragment, cell membranes bleb but do not burst, and cellular contents are not released. The dead cells undergo rapid phagocytosis without an inflammatory response. In addition to the morphologic differences between necrotic cell death and apoptosis, a characteristic process of DNA degradation by cellular proteases occurs. This DNA degradation is recognized by isolating cellular DNA and running it out on a gel, revealing a laddering of DNA pieces of various sizes.

One of the first and best characterized examples of programmed cell death was in the worm, *C. elegans,* in which exactly 131 cells die during development at specific times and in specific places in a genetically controlled fashion. Some of the genes responsible for this process have been cloned and characterized in the worm and mammalian counterparts identified. Additional positive and negative regulators of programmed cell death have been discovered and given innovative names such as reaper and death domain. It is clear that programmed cell death is important in mammalian development, in tissue homeostasis, in immune-mediated cell death, and in the dysregulation

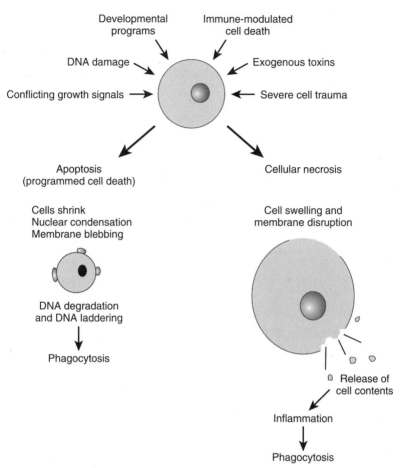

FIGURE 3–9. **Programmed Cell Death—Apoptosis.** A number of processes, listed on the left of the figure, can induce apoptosis. This form of cell death contrasts with necrotic cell death in several major features. Cells shrink rather than swell, and inflammation is involved in the phagocytic process.

of cell growth associated with cancer. Indeed the programmed cell death system has been identified as a target for gene therapy in cancer. The role of programmed cell death in cancer and its regulation by events associated with the cell cycle is discussed in Chapter 7. It is clear from the rapidly expanding literature on programmed cell death that regulation of cell death will prove to be as complex and important as regulation of cell proliferation.

It is now recognized that a number of neurodegenerative diseases are associated with neuronal cell loss not involving inflammation and therefore likely to be due to programmed cell death. Although the complexity of the process has prevented investigators from defining how programmed cell death is responsible for neuronal loss in ALS, the potential of altering the balance of positive and negative cell death genes, of interfering with their function, or of altering the redox state of neuronal cells holds hope for the future therapy of ALS.

## SUGGESTED READING

### Finding the Amyotrophic Lateral Sclerosis Gene

Deng H-X, Hentati A, Tainer JA, et al: Amyotrophic lateral sclerosis and structural defects in Cu, Zn superoxide dismutase. Science 261:1047–1051, 1993.

Rosen DR, Siddique T, Patterson D, et al: Mutations in Cu/Zn superoxide dismutase gene are associated with familial amyotrophic lateral sclerosis. Nature 362:59–62, 1993.

Weissenbach J, Gyapay G, Dib C, et al: A second-generation linkage map of the human genome. Nature 359:794–801, 1992.

### Amyotropic Lateral Sclerosis Is a Gain of Function Disease

Brown RH: Amyotrophic lateral sclerosis: Recent insights from genetics and transgenic mice. Cell 80:687–692, 1995.

Gurney ME, Pu H, Chiu AY, et al: Motor neuron degeneration in mice that express a human Cu, Zn superoxide dismutase mutation. Science 264:1772–1775, 1994.

### Apoptosis and Amyotrophic Lateral Sclerosis

Bellamy COC, Malcomson RDG, Harrison DJ, et al: Cell death in health and disease: The biology and regulation of apoptosis. Semin Cancer Biol 6:3–16, 1995.

Greenlund LJS, Deckwerth TL, Johnson EM: Superoxide dismutase delays neuronal apoptosis: A role for reactive oxygen species in programmed neuronal cell death. Neuron 14:303–315, 1995.

Rabizadeh S, Butler Gralla E, Borchelt DR, et al: Mutations associated with amyotrophic lateral sclerosis convert superoxide dismutase from an antiapoptotic gene to a proapoptotic gene: Studies in yeast and neural cells. Proc Natl Acad Sci USA 92:3024–3028, 1995.

Steller H: Mechanisms and genes of cellular suicide. Science 267:1445–1448, 1995.

# Alveolar Proteinosis in the Adult and Newborn: A Knockout Surprise and a Surfactant Gene Mutation

embryonic stem cells • homologous recombination • targeted mutations • gene knockouts • knockins • restriction fragment length polymorphisms • Cre-lox

Pulmonary alveolar proteinosis (PAP) is a rare disease that was first described in 1958. It presents as an alveolar pattern pulmonary infiltrate on chest radiographs; there are nonspecific symptoms, including dyspnea, and a protracted course, often with spontaneous remissions. Although no causative agent has been identified, PAP has been reported in association with hematologic malignancies, immunocompromised states, and accelerated silicosis. The alveoli are filled with proteinaceous material that is rich in phospholipids and surfactant proteins. Animal models have provided no insight as to its cause, although it has been noted that rats exposed to various inorganic dusts such as silica have a similar picture.

Although the cause remains unclear, it is now generally thought that PAP results from an imbalance of pulmonary surfactant production and secretion versus surfactant clearance and recycling. Alveolar macrophages in PAP appear to be functionally deficient, suggesting that the defect may lie in the surfactant clearance pathway. Recently, molecular biology has provided insights into two possible mechanisms responsible for the accumulation of proteinaceous material in alveoli that characterizes alveolar proteinosis. One relates to abnormalities in *SPB* associated with congenital alveolar proteinosis (CAP), which is a uniformly fatal disease of the full-term newborn. Recently a mutation in the *SPB* gene has been described in association with CAP. A second model of PAP relates to a surprise phenotype in mice in whom the gene for granulocyte-macrophage colony stimulating factor (GM-CSF) has been "knocked out." In the absence of *GM-CSF*, at 2 to 3 months of age mice begin to accumulate amorphous, acellular material in the alveolar space that is rich in surfactant lipoprotein and has the morphologic and biochemical abnormalities described in PAP.

The studies describing the PAP model were actually begun in order to more clearly define the functions of GM-CSF. GM-CSF is a cytokine that plays a role in regulating hematopoietic cell proliferation and differentiation and has been shown to have a number of other diverse functions in various model systems. To better define GM-CSF function, investigators used a form of gene targeting that allows one to introduce a known mutation into a specific gene or, in this case, to completely eliminate or knock out a gene of interest. The result of this targeted *GM-CSF* knockout was an animal model of PAP.

## Targeted Gene Expression: Knockouts and Determining the Function of a Gene

Knocking out a gene or targeting a mutation to a gene in an animal is not a simple or an inexpensive task. One can overexpress a mutated gene in a cell or a transgenic animal, but overexpression by itself does not necessarily eliminate the normal gene and its function. In the past several years, the technique of gene knockout, that is, eliminating a gene, has become a standard method for defining gene function. It has been used to create animal models of cystic fibrosis and a number of other diseases and has proved to be extremely valuable in dissecting the role of various regulators of development in the embryo.

Homologous recombination is the focal point of a number of important concepts in molecular biology, and the events associated with homologous recombination are fundamental to many molecular biologic methods such as the targeted gene expression that is used to create gene knockouts. Homologous recombination occurs normally with relatively high frequency during the meiotic cell divisions that lead to the formation of male and female germ cells (Fig. 4–1). Each sperm and each egg contains 23 chromosomes, which represent the genetic material contributed by each parent. Sperm and egg unite to form the zygote, which contains 46 chromosomes—23 male and 23 female. Two meiotic cell divisions follow, during which genetic material is transferred between chromosomes, and each germ line cell ends up with 23 single rather than 23 paired chromosomes. Somatic cells contain 23 pairs of chromosomes and thus are diploid cells. They undergo mitotic rather than meiotic cell division. During the first meiotic cell division, maternal and paternal chromosomes are duplicated, forming a cell that contains 46 male and 46 female chromosomes. During prophase of the first meiotic division, homologous male and female chromosomes line up, attach briefly, and exchange portions of their DNA. This process is called crossing over, and the cutting and ligating of opposite pieces of DNA is called homologous recombination (see Chapter 3). There are, on average, three such recombination events per meiotic division on each chromosome, and these events are responsible for much of the genetic variation among individuals of similar genetic background. The next meiotic division occurs without DNA synthesis, and germ line cells return to their haploid, 23-chromosome state.

Although homologous recombination occurs with relatively high frequency during meiotic cell division, it also occurs at low frequency in mitotic cell divisions in somatic cells, such as the embryonic stem (ES) cells. During mitotic recombination of ES cells, mutant DNA constructs can be inserted exactly in the right spot on the chromosome to replace normal DNA. The trick in creating knockout mice is to select only those ES cells that have the mutated gene inserted in place of the normal gene.

Figures 4–2 and 4–3 illustrate the basic steps involved in creating a knockout mouse. A mutated gene is made, inserted in a vector, and transfected into ES cells. ES cells are pluripotential cells removed from the blastocyst that can be kept in an undifferentiated state in the appropriate media on a fibroblast feeder layer. When the in vitro growth conditions are altered, these cells have the potential of differentiating into virtually any cell type in the body. ES cells are obtained from the blastocyst of one pregnant female. A mutated gene is inserted to replace the normal gene in the ES cells, and those cells with the mutated gene are selected by one of those clever molecular biologic tricks, which is described further on. These cells are then introduced into the blastocyst of another pseudopregnant mouse, where the ES cells containing the mutated gene contribute to all tissues of the mouse, creating a chimera (an animal whose cells contain foreign DNA as well as their own DNA). Heterozygous males and females are then bred to produce homozygotes that exclusively express the mutated (interrupted) gene rather than the normal gene of interest. The methods used to produce gene knockout mice are based on important genetic concepts such as homologous recombination, on the basic biology of ES cells, and on techniques that

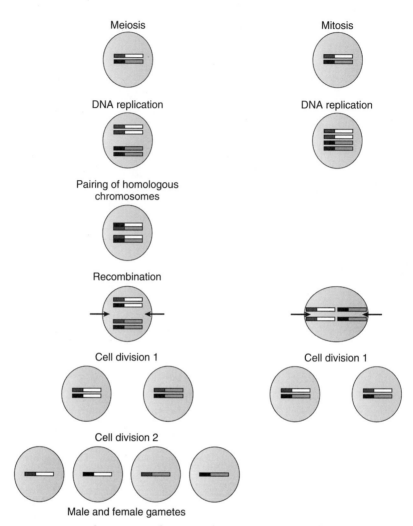

FIGURE 4–1. **Homologous Recombination.** There are two types of cell division: meiotic and mitotic. Meiosis generates the male and female germ cells (gametes) that carry, on 23 unpaired chromosomes, the genetic information to be transmitted to new generations. Meiosis involves two cell divisions but only one round of DNA synthesis, thus producing cells with only one set of either male or female chromosomes. During the first meiotic cell division, male and female chromosomes align and exchange pieces of DNA from homologous parts of the chromosomes. In this figure, the male (*dark gray cross-hatched*) chromosomes exchange a piece of DNA (*solid, cross-hatched*) with a piece of DNA (*lighter gray stippled*) on the female (*white*) chromosome. This homologous recombination results in the insertion of a piece of the male chromosome in exactly the correct position on a chromosome in the female germ cell and vice versa. This phenomenon occurs at a much lower frequency during subsequent mitotic cell divisions of somatic cells. In the example on the right, the gray stippled piece of the female chromosome does not recombine with the male chromosome. Mitotic recombination is the basis of embryonic stem (ES) cell recombination for the targeted gene mutations involved in creating gene knock-outs.

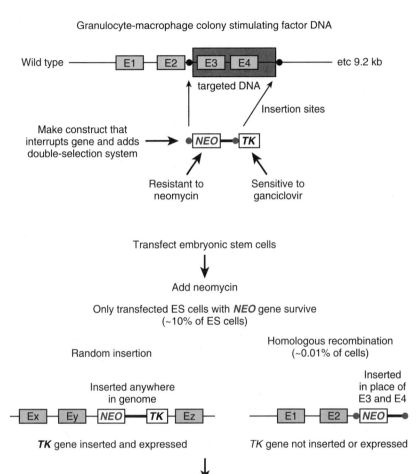

FIGURE 4–2. **Gene Knockout: Targeted Insertion of DNA.** A piece of DNA containing the *NEO* gene, which conveys resistance to the toxic effects of the antibiotic neomycin to those cells that have been transfected, is targeted to exchange, via homologous recombination, with exons 3 and 4 (*E3* and *E4*) plus a small portion of intronic DNA (*darker shaded box*). The piece of DNA has insertion sites (*gray circles*) that are identical to sequences that bracket the piece of DNA to be replaced (*black circles*). If the construct is inserted in a random fashion, that is, any place other than the targeted site (in the example, between *Ey* and *Ez*) the thymidine kinase gene (*TK*), which is part of the original construct, will also be inserted. On the addition of ganciclovir, cells expressing the *TK* gene are killed (see text for explanation). If the construct replaces the targeted exons, the *TK* gene is not included, and the cells that recombine in this homologous fashion survive the addition of ganciclovir.

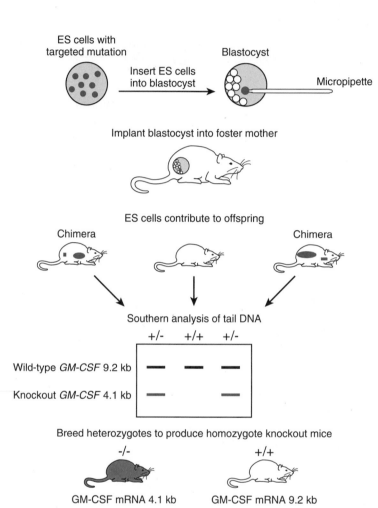

FIGURE 4–3. **Gene Knockout: Making the Mouse.** ES cells that contain the targeted mutation described in Figure 4–2 are inserted via micropipette into a blastocyst taken from a pregnant mouse, and this blastocyst is then placed into the uterus of a foster mother. The blastocyst contains cells from a mouse with a coat color that differs from that of the ES cell strain. Thus, chimeric offspring (offspring expressing both the ES cell genes and the blastocyst genes) have a mixed-color coat. Southern blots of the DNA extracted from the tails of the offspring reveal whether they express only normal or normal plus targeted *GM-CSF* DNA. The heterozygous mice are bred to produce homozygous *GM-CSF* knockout mice.

allow selection of those cells in which the normal gene has been replaced by a mutated gene.

To create the knockout mice that acquired PAP, the wild-type *GM-CSF* gene is disrupted by placing a construct containing a neomycin resistance gene minus exons 3 and 4 after exon 2 of the *GM-CSF* gene (see Fig. 4–2). Since this insert eliminates the subsequent exons, it prevents transcription of the complete gene. The ES cells are then transfected with this construct and grown in the presence of neomycin. Only those cells that incorporate the vector into their genome and express the neomycin resistance gene survive. This first selection step eliminates all nontransfected cells. The viral thymidine kinase (*TK*) gene is placed at the end of the mutant construct for double selection. This second selection ensures that only those cells with the mutant construct inserted in place of the normal gene via homologous recombination survive. During homologous recombination, the mutant gene replaces the homologous segment in the normal gene, with the neomycin resistance gene sandwiched in. The herpesvirus promoter and *TK* gene, being at the end of the artificial construct, lie outside the matching sequences at the recombination site, and this segment of the mutated gene is not integrated into the chromosome. Once separated from the rest of the construct, the *TK* gene is degraded. In contrast, at sites of random insertion (the far more frequent event), the whole construct is inserted and integrated into the chromosome at a single site so that the *TK* gene is expressed. This gene produces an enzyme that converts the drug ganciclovir to a purine analog that can compete with normal purine nucleotides for incorporation into DNA during cell proliferation. However, it cannot be used for DNA synthesis, so cells expressing the *TK* gene in the presence of ganciclovir die. In the presence of ganciclovir, those cells expressing *TK* (which occurs only with random insertions) are killed. The cells that have inserted the construct by homologous recombination replacing the normal gene fail to incorporate the *TK* gene at the end of construct and are not killed by ganciclovir; they are therefore the only cells to survive the double selection process.

The ES cells that survive the double selection process and thus have no translatable *GM-CSF*, are then microinjected into a blastocyst taken from a pregnant donor. The blastocyst, containing the "knockout" ES cells, is inserted into a foster mother and an embryo develops, with mutant ES cells contributing to the formation of many tissues. A male and a female heterozygote ( +/− for the mutation), each with the mutant gene (knockout) on one allele, are mated. Homozygotes ( −/− ) that result from this mating are true knockout mice. If the coat color of the blastocyst donor is different from that of the ES cell lineage, animals expressing genes from both lineages will have a two-color coat, helping to identify chimeric mice.

*GM-CSF* −/− knockout mice produced by this method developed a pulmonary picture resembling PAP, with excess surfactant lipids and proteins in the alveolar lavage but normal amounts of surfactant protein mRNA expressed in the lungs. Immunocytochemical analysis revealed normal amounts of SPA in type 2 cells but increased amounts of SPA in alveolar macrophages. These findings suggest that the defect in this model of PAP lies not in overproduction but in altered clearance of surfactant, presumably by alveolar macrophages. The absence of *GM-CSF* in knockout mice may alter macrophage functions such as binding, uptake, or degradation of surfactant, resulting in accumulation of this material in the alveolus with the appearance of the clinical syndrome of PAP. It is known that type 2 cells normally produce and secrete *GM-CSF*, and thus may regulate a number of alveolar macrophage functions. This knockout surprise has provided a number of insights into the pathogenesis of PAP and can now serve as a model for testing macrophage–type 2 cell interactions and possible new approaches to the treatment of PAP.

## Replacing One Gene with Another: "Knockin Mice"

One of the problems of writing this book has been the incredible rate at which molecular biologic discoveries are being made and new methods and concepts are being developed. In the last stages of writing this chapter, knockins, the partner of knockouts, appeared. In this case, the idea is to replace a gene that been eliminated with another gene to see if it can substitute for the function of the knocked-out gene. Comparing a knockout model of gene 1 to a knockout model of gene 2 does not provide that information because gene 1 and gene 2 may be expressed in different cells at different times in development or they may respond to different regulatory factors. Enter gene knockins, that is, replacing a gene that is knocked out by a different gene that is regulated in exactly the same fashion as the gene that has been knocked out.

In the article describing this technique, two similar but not identical genes that code for transcription factors (see Chapter 8) and are normally expressed at slightly different times in different parts of the brain were compared. When one gene *(En-1)* is knocked out, a large portion of the midbrain does not form and the embryos die. When *En-2* is knocked out, parts of the cerebellum do not form, but the mice are viable. The question to be answered was, do the proteins encoded by these two genes serve different functions or is the difference in knockout results of the two genes explained by different timing and position of their expression. The approach (Fig. 4–4) was to knock out *En-1* in a standard fashion, but to do so with a construct that when inserted into the correct position replaces *En-1* with the cDNA for *En-2*. *En-2* is now driven by the *En-1* promoter and should be expressed at the same time and in the same places as the now absent *En-1*. If *En-2* serves the same function as *En-1*, the mice will live and form midbrains; if it does not "rescue" the *En-1* knockout, the animals will not have mid- and hindbrains and will die. The experiment worked; when *En-1* was knocked out and replaced by *En-2*, the animals lived. Thus, the proteins

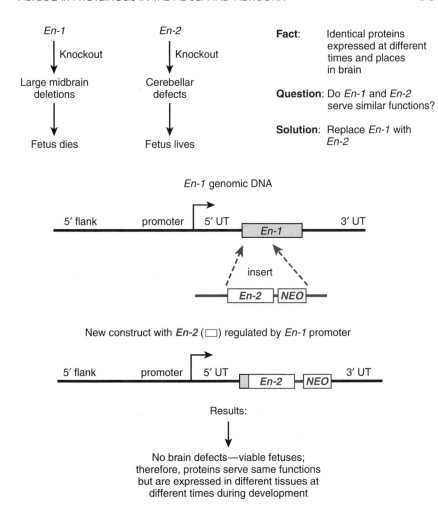

FIGURE 4–4. **Gene Knockin: Replacing One Gene with Another.** In this experiment, the question was whether the En-1 and En-2 proteins serve the same functions. The *En-2* gene is inserted by homologous recombination into the *En-1* site, disrupting *En-1* with the *En-2* DNA. In homozygotes, the *En-2* gene is now driven by the regulatory regions of *En-1*. Thus En-2 is expressed at the times and in the places that *En-1* is normally expressed, effectively replacing *En-1*.

serve similar functions, and the difference between them results from their different patterns of expression. This method also has great potential for defining the functions of genes and determining the functions of portions of the proteins encoded by these genes because one can replace a knocked-out gene by the same gene that has been altered to change only one part of the encoded protein or to have one specific mutation.

## Conditional Knockouts: Cre-Lox

One of the problems with knocking out an important gene is that it often results in a lethal mutation, that is, the gene is so important to the development of the early embryo that the embryo does not form and no specific phenotype is defined. The solution would be to excise the gene at a point after the embryo has formed or to create the knockout in the tissue of interest without disrupting function in any other tissue. One can certainly express genes in a tissue-specific fashion, for example, by using the SPC promoter to target gene expression in type 2 cells (see Chapter 8) or the fatty acid binding protein promoter to target a gene to the intestine (see Chapter 6). However, targeting gene knockout in time or place is much more difficult. Recently, a clever new method for accomplishing this task was described. As is often the case, the method uses bacterial genetics in a mammalian system.

The method, site-directed recombination, or conditional gene targeting, uses the Cre-loxP system. The Cre recombinase is a bacterial enzyme that recognizes a specific 34–base pair nucleotide sequence (loxP) that flanks a segment of DNA. The "flanked by lox" segment of DNA is called flox. Cre cuts the loxP sites, excises the intervening DNA, and recombines the cut ends of DNA (Fig. 4–5). The loxP sites can be inserted into the genome using the ES cell homologous recombination techniques with antibiotic selection that was detailed earlier. The flox gene animals are then bred with Cre-expressing transgenic mice. When Cre meets flox, the flanked DNA segment is excised and a gene knockout occurs. If Cre is driven by a universal promoter such as the cytomegalovirus promoter, it will be expressed in all cells and it will excise the loxP flanked gene in all cells of the gamete. The resultant gene excision is no different from the usual gene-targeting knockout. However, if the Cre transgenic mouse expresses Cre in certain cells only, gene knockout will occur only in those cells or tissues that express Cre. Cre transgenic mice expressing Cre in only T or B lymphocytes have already been developed, and it is only a matter of time before other tissue-specific transgenic models will become available; Cre driven by SPC would provide an experimental system in which critical genes could be eliminated only in SPC–expressing cells. An equally powerful experimental system would be one in which the gene of interest could be knocked out at a precise point in time. A Cre transgenic mouse with an interferon-inducible promoter has been produced. Cre is not expressed until interferon is given. In mice that have been crossed with targeted loxP sites, the flox gene is excised in those cells or tissues that respond to interferon. Preliminary results have shown that not all tissues respond to interferon. It is likely that one will eventually be able to eliminate a gene at a specific time in a specific cell or tissue.

Another conditional gene induction-elimination model was recently developed. In this system, the gene of interest, not normally expressed or expressed at low levels in a cell, is transfected in a vector that includes a tetracycline response element. In the absence of tetracycline, the gene is not

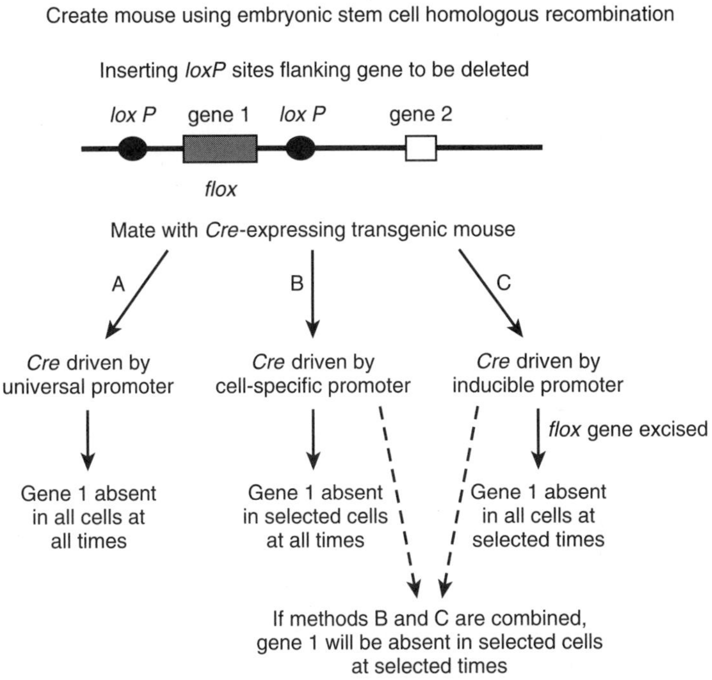

FIGURE 4–5. **Conditional Gene Knockouts: Knockouts When and Where You Want Them with Cre-loxP.** Lox P sites are inserted around the gene to be eliminated using ES cell technology. The gene flanked by lox P is called flox or flanked by lox. The resulting mice are then mated with transgenic mice expressing the *Cre* gene. If *Cre* is expressed in every cell, it will recognize the *loxP* sites and cut out the *flox* gene in all cells at conception. If *Cre* is expressed via a cell-specific promoter, *flox* will be eliminated only in those cells expressing *Cre*. If *Cre* is driven by an inducible promoter, it will be expressed and will cut out the *flox* gene only when induced, for example, by a hormone. Thus, the function of a gene in a specific cell or at a specific time can be assessed.

expressed. When tetracycline is provided, the gene is induced in a concentration-dependent fashion. This system has been employed in a number of cell lines, using usual transfection methods, and can be adapted for use in transgenic mice. The method is especially useful in defining the functions of genes that may be toxic to cells or that create growth disadvantages to cells that express the gene when normal transfection methods are used. A tetracycline repressor can also be used to conditionally turn off transfected genes.

## Congenital Alveolar Proteinosis (CAP): *SPB* Is the Key

The clinical syndrome of CAP has been recognized for a number of years. It presents in full-term rather than premature infants, with a physiologic picture somewhat similar to the respiratory distress syndrome of immaturity but with a pathologic picture of protein-filled alveoli that is similar to PAP. The disease is uniformly fatal. In 1993, a group of investigators described two siblings with CAP who had no SPB protein in their lung lavage or lung tissue and no SPB mRNA in Northern blots of lung tissue biopsy specimens. In contrast, both SPA and SPC mRNA and proteins were abundant. Subsequently, similar cases were described, the autosomal recessive nature of the disease established, the defective production of SPB confirmed, and a mutation in the *SPB* gene identified. The human *SPB* gene has been cloned and sequenced, its regulation has begun to be characterized (see Chapter 8), and attempts to transfect rat lungs with the human *SPB* gene have been reported. However, attempts to treat infants with CAP using natural surfactant that contains *SPB* have failed. The whole experiment has moved rapidly, although the explanation for the mutation and the cause of the PAP-like disease itself, with the lack of surfactant clearance from the alveoli, is still incomplete.

The fact that *SPB* was deficient in several cases of CAP and that the disease tends to be familial first suggested that a genetic defect was causal. To determine if there was a mutation in the *SPB* gene, RNA was isolated from lung biopsy specimens of CAP patients, was reverse transcribed into cDNA, and the cDNA was amplified with primers that covered several regions of the human *SPB* gene. The resultant polymerase chain reaction products were cloned and then sequenced. As illustrated in Figure 4–5, an insertion of two base pairs and a change in a third base pair was found at site 375 of the cDNA, in codon 121, which is in exon 4 of the 3'-untranslated region of the gene. This insertion of GAA for a C in codon 121 produced a frameshift mutation (see Fig 3–4), with insertion of several premature stop codons farther downstream in the open reading frame of the *SPB* gene in exons 6 and 7. The result was that the insertion and frameshift mutation ensured that SPB mRNA was not translated after codon 214 and no SPB protein was made. The insertion is illustrated in Figure 4–6. The frameshift mutation also introduced a change in restriction enzyme cutting sites, adding a new *SfuI* (TT/CGAA) and a *TagI* (T/CGA) site that resulted in the diagnostic restriction fragment length polymorphisms shown in Figure 4–5. The mutation also resulted in an unstable SPB mRNA so that even the mutant mRNA was not seen on Northern blots of lung tissue.

Much remains to be learned of the biologic role that *SPB* plays in surfactant processing and what goes wrong in the absence of *SPB* to produce CAP. In addition, abnormalities may appear in the processing of SPC proteins, implying that *SPB* itself is involved in the function of other surfactant proteins. Recently an *SPB* knockout mouse was reported using methods similar to those described earlier. These animals died at birth with no SPB protein and abnormal SPC protein, type 2 cells that lack lamellar bodies, and an absence of tubular myelin in alveoli. The knockout mice did not have the pathologic picture of CAP, but this may be due to the fact that they died immediately after birth. Finally, at least one infant with CAP has been reported with a

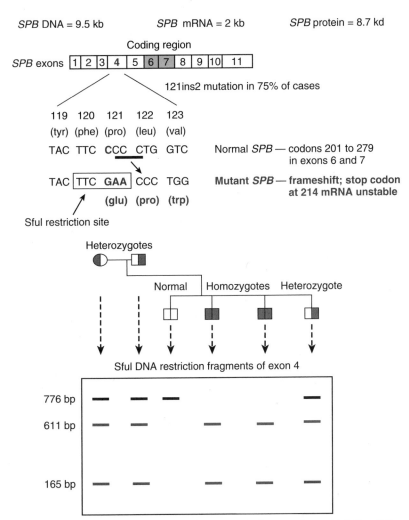

FIGURE 4–6. **A Mutation in the *SPB* Gene (121ins2) That Results in CAP.** The *SPB* gene has 11 exons that produce a 2-kb mRNA and an 8.7-kd protein. Exons 6 and 7 contain the coding region (open reading frame) for *SPB*. The main mutation described in CAP patients occurs in exon 4 of the 5'-untranslated region. The first C of this codon (**in gray**) is mutated to a G and an AA is also inserted, resulting in a GAA instead of a CCC codon. The result is a glutamine instead of a proline amino acid. The two inserted nucleotides also produce a frameshift that results in a stop signal at codon 214 of exon 6. No complete SPB protein is produced, and the SPB that is produced is rapidly degraded. The 121ins2 mutation creates a new restriction site for the enzyme Sflu, which cuts between TT and CCGAA at codons 120 and 121 to create a diagnostic test for the mutation. Heterozygotes have one normal allele of 776 base pairs and one abnormal allele with restriction sites that produce fragments of 611 and 165 base pairs. Homozygotes, who manifest CAP, have only the abnormal restriction fragments.

normal *SPB* gene, suggesting that other causes of CAP may exist. All this work has occurred within the past 2 years, illustrating the rapid movement from test tube or vector to bedside that has characterized the application of molecular biology to clinical medicine. The observation of *SPB* deficiency in CAP has prompted new studies examining other cases of neonatal respiratory distress and new attempts at gene therapy for surfactant proteins.

## SUGGESTED READING

### Granulocyte-Macrophage Colony Stimulating Factor Knockout

Dranoff G, Crawford AD, Sadelain M, et al: Involvement of granulocyte-macrophage colony stimulating factor in pulmonary homeostasis. Science 264:713–716, 1994.

Huffman JA, Hull WM, Dranoff G, et al: Pulmonary epithelial cell expression of GM-CSF corrects the alveolar proteinosis in GM-CSF–deficient mice. J Clin Invest 97:649–655, 1996.

### Targeted Gene Replacement: The Concept

Capecchi MR: Targeted gene replacement. Sci Am March, 52–59, 1994.

Hanks M, Wurst W, Anson-Cartwright L, et al: Rescue of the EN-1 mutant phenotype by replacement of En-1 with En-2. Science 269:679–682, 1995.

Melton D: Gene targeting in the mouse. Bioessays 16:633–637, 1994.

### Conditional Gene Targeting: The Cre-Lox System

Gossen M, Freundlieb S, Bender G, et al: Transcriptional activation by tetracyclines in mammalian cells. Science 268:1766–1769, 1995.

Kuhn R, Schenk F, Aguet M, et al: Inducible gene targeting in mice. Science 269:1427–1429, 1995.

Rajewsky K, Gu H, Kuhn R, et al: Conditional gene targeting. J Clin Invest 98(Suppl):S51–S53, 1996.

### *SPB* and Hereditary Alveolar Proteinosis

Clark JC, Wert SA, Bachurski CJ, et al: Targeted disruption of the surfactant protein B gene disrupts surfactant homeostasis, causing respiratory failure in newborn mice. Proc Natl Acad Sci USA 92:7794–7798, 1995.

Nogee LM, De Mello DE, Dehner LP, et al: Brief report: Deficiency of pulmonary surfactant B in congenital alveolar proteinosis. N Engl J Med 328:406–409, 1993.

Nogee LM, Garnier G, Dieetz HC, et al: A mutation in the surfactant protein B gene responsible for fatal neonatal respiratory disease in multiple kindreds. J Clin Invest 93:1860–1863, 1994.

# $\alpha_1$-Antitrypsin Deficiency: The Perfect Disease for Gene Therapy

protein structure • gene therapy • viral vectors

Gene therapy is one of the most exciting applications of molecular biology to human disease and certainly one that has captured the imagination of the public, the hopes of patients with both genetic and acquired diseases, and the money of venture capitalists. $\alpha_1$-Antitrypsin (AAT) deficiency and cystic fibrosis have led the way in advancing the basic science of gene therapy and in the number of clinical trials being carried out.

The explosion in human gene therapy began in earnest about 5 years ago when approval was given to replace the defective gene in a patient with congenital adenosine deaminase deficiency. This enzyme is essential to the immune system; individuals without the enzyme are susceptible to a variety of infections and usually die at an early age. The first gene transfer experiments were ex vivo, that is, the gene was transfected into cells in culture and the cells were then infused into the patients. The cloning of the cystic fibrosis transmembrane regulator (*CFTR*)—first in in vitro experiments, then in vivo animal trials, and finally in human experiments, providing normal *CFTR* to patients with cystic fibrosis, appeared on the front pages of scientific and lay publications. The cure for cystic fibrosis seemed to be just around the corner, and the era of gene therapy for human genetic diseases had arrived. This was the high point of the public's romance with gene therapy.

Over the past year or two, the picture has changed and changed dramatically. Getting missing or mutant genes into the right cells and expressing them in a stable fashion has not proved easy. The first full report of *CFTR* transfections in cystic fibrosis patients has shown low levels of gene transfer and no correction of the epithelial ion transport defect. In response to a growing number of questions about the lack of clear-cut success with gene therapy despite large expenditures of public and private money, the National Institutes of Health has set up a number of committees to review the status of gene therapy, the problems investigators face, and the directions new research should take. A special news report in a recent issue of *Science* discussed the growing awareness that ideal systems for delivering genes to cells and tissues are far from realization.

This chapter reviews the theory behind gene therapy, some of the technical issues that have limited its effectiveness, and some of its exciting potential. Gene therapy is discussed further in Chapters 6 and 7. The review of gene therapy in *Science* pointed out that the majority of approved clinical trials of gene therapy have been for acquired diseases such as cancer and human immunodeficiency virus (HIV) rather than hereditary diseases. However, if one had to pick a genetic disease to start with, AAT deficiency would be near the top of the list.

The goal in AAT deficiency is a simple one: the production of sufficient amounts of a circulating molecule without the need to target the gene to a specific tissue. Although the disease to be prevented is primarily in the lung, the protein is produced in the liver and released into the circulation. Individuals who have greater than 30 to 40% of the normal level of AAT do not have clinically apparent disease, so low levels of gene expression will be protective. Although the defective protein may cause liver disease in patients with low levels of normal AAT, one usually does not have to worry about the effects of the mutant molecule; all that is necessary is a source of circulating AAT. As will be seen, even in this conceptually easy to treat genetic disease, success has eluded gene therapists. The reasons this has happened explain a great deal about the basics of gene therapy.

## $\alpha_1$-Antitrypsin Deficiency: The Disease and the Defect

It was only 30 years ago that the link between AAT deficiency and emphysema was made by Laurell and Ericksson. During this ensuing period, the biochemistry of the molecule, the pathophysiology of the disease, and the genetic basis of the AAT mutation and its effect on protein structure have been defined, and protein replacement and trials of gene therapy are in progress.

With the power of molecular biology, the progress has been incredibly rapid, surpassed perhaps only by the pace of research in cystic fibrosis.

AAT is one member of the large family of serine protease inhibitors. Its main target is neutrophil elastase, which cleaves and then binds AAT, inactivating the enzyme and forming a complex that is removed from the circulation by the liver. The gene for AAT is on chromosome 14 at the 14q32.1 locus. The gene is 12.2 kb long; the mRNA is 1.4 kb in the liver and slightly longer in monocytes, coding for a 52-kd secreted protein that is heavily glycosylated and thus is post-translationally modified. Its major site of production is the liver. The gene has two promoters, one that is specific for monocytes and one that is specific for the liver. There are at least 75 different AAT alleles designated Pi or protease inhibitor types, although only a few are associated with disease. The normal allele is called M, and the two most common mutant alleles in Europe and the United States are Z and S. Clinically apparent emphysema, the AAT deficiency phenotype, does not occur unless circulating AAT levels are less than 20% of normal. This happens only in individuals who are Pi ZZ homozygotes or have null mutations (Pi null), in which no AAT protein is produced. Pi MZ heterozygotes have intermediate levels of AAT and do not acquire clinically apparent disease. Pi SS individuals also have intermediate levels of AAT and do not acquire clinical disease. Pi ZZ and Pi null individuals have decreased survival, the chances of being alive at age 60 years being 20% versus 85% in normal persons, even without smoking as a factor. Smoking markedly widens the gap between normal individuals and AAT-deficient persons.

Before the biologic characteristics of the AAT Pi Z mutation are discussed, the concept of protein folding and the formation of tertiary protein structure must be presented. As discussed in Chapter 1, proteins consist of a series of amino acids coded for by the three-letter mRNA codons. The amino acids link together by hydrogen bonds to form a peptide chain with an amino terminus and a carboxyl terminus (Fig. 5–1). However, proteins rarely exist as simple chains of amino acids. Bonds form between amino acid side chains as a result of noncovalent (weak) or covalent (strong) interactions between individual amino acids. These interactions result in the peptides assuming first a secondary folded structure and then a tertiary three-dimensional structure. Three major tertiary structures exist: coiled α-helices, closely packed linear chains that form β-sheets, and tightly packed globular proteins. Many proteins like AAT consist of combinations of these tertiary structures.

The Z mutation is a simple point mutation, a substitution of an A for a G at codon 342. The result of this single base pair substitution is a change at position 342 of a negatively charged glutamic acid to a positively charged lysine. The charge attraction between amino acids at position 342 and 290 is replaced by charge-repelling amino acids, and the bend in the tertiary structure of the protein at this site (at the reactive center of the protein) is altered (Fig. 5–2). This bend and the 342–290 bond normally introduces an α-helix between two β-sheets of the protein. The Pi Z mutation of glutamic acid to

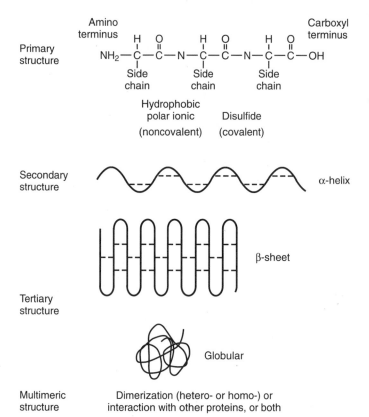

Peptide backbone of individual amino acids

FIGURE 5–1. **Protein Structure.** The three-dimensional structure that a protein assumes has a profound effect on its functions. Proteins are made up of chains of individual amino acids that are linked together by peptide bonds between a carbon and a nitrogen of each amino acid. The side chains depicted under primary structure represent the individual amino acids that interact via noncovalent or covalent bonding to produce changes in shape that confer secondary and three-dimensional tertiary structure to the protein. As an example, amino acids such as lysine and histidine are basic and bind via charge attraction to amino acids such as aspartic acid or glutamic acid. Guided by these interactions, peptide chains fold into helices or form sheets or globular structures. These various secondary folded shapes then interact to form three-dimensional combinations that determine the final shape of the protein, providing active sites for enzymes, binding sites for extracellular matrix molecules, interactions with DNA or specific receptors, and other types of interactions. Some proteins form functional units by interacting with another molecule of the same protein (two such proteins form homodimers), with molecules of a different protein (two such proteins form heterodimers), or with several of the same or other proteins, forming multimers.

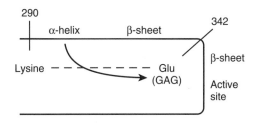

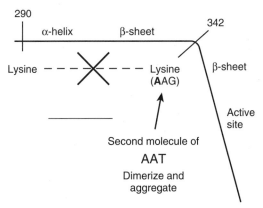

FIGURE 5–2. **AAT: the Pi Z Mutation and Its Effect on Tertiary Structure.** Glutamic acid (+) at position 342 sits at a crucial bend in AAT close to the active site for interaction with neutrophil elastase. Glutamic acid and lysine (−) at position 290 form a bridge. In the AAT Pi Z mutation, a point mutation substituting an A for a G at 342 results in a lysine instead of glutamic acid. The charge attraction between 342 and 290 is abolished, and the bend at 342 does not occur. As the molecule opens up, another molecule of AAT is now free to dimerize with the first molecule, leading to aggregation of the AAT protein in the endoplasmic reticulum. However, the active site is not affected by the aggregation.

lysine prevents the introduction of the helix between two sheets, the bend in the protein at 342 does not occur, and the two sheets open to allow dimerization with another AAT molecule. Dimerization leads to aggregation of AAT in the endoplasmic reticulum, preventing its secretion. The mutant AAT has virtually normal antielastase activity, but because of the aggregation noted earlier, it is not secreted. The accumulation of AAT in the endoplasmic reticulum results in liver disease in approximately 10% of infants with the ZZ phenotype and liver function abnormalities in 50% of Pi ZZ adults. Pi S also involves a point mutation in which a glutamic acid at position 264 is replaced by a valine, altering another bridge between 264 and a lysine at 387. However, this mutation does not appear to influence protein folding or elastase inhibition, and secreted levels of AAT are only mildly reduced. In null mutations, a variety of deletions or mutations results in premature stop codons, with the result that no stable AAT protein is produced, and therefore AAT levels are zero.

## Gene Therapy in $\alpha_1$-Antitrypsin Deficiency: The Goal

Since the liver disease in AAT usually is not a problem, the goal of therapy has been to ignore the appearance of the mutant protein in the liver and to focus on providing sufficient AAT to reach circulating levels that are greater than 10 to 20% of normal, above which clinical lung disease does not occur. The approaches to this goal have ranged from putting the gene in the liver, the lungs, or the skeletal muscle cells to using the peritoneum as a surface for implanting AAT-producing cells. Since the goal has been to increase circulating levels of AAT, investigators have not worried about normal regulation of the gene; rather, they have generally used strong constitutive promoters that result in constant production of AAT. To date, they have come close but have not yet achieved their goals. The problem has not been in expressing the AAT gene nor in producing circulating protein, rather it has been the problem that has affected virtually all forms of gene treatment of hereditary diseases—the inability to produce high levels of persistent expression without the need for repeated gene transfections. To understand this problem, a general discussion of gene therapy is in order before one can focus on the technical problems that have led to the reassessment of gene therapy noted at the beginning of this chapter.

There are several important questions that must be answered before one deals with the all-important practical issue of which vector to use for the actual gene transfer.

### WHICH CELL TO TRANSFECT?

Concerns about the transfer of viral genes from the recipient to subsequent generations have limited transfections to somatic rather than germ cells. Germ cells, sperm and eggs, will pass the transfected genes to all cells that derive from subsequent matings; in somatic cells, the transfected gene appears only in the transfected cell and in its daughter cells and therefore will not be passed on to subsequent generations. In some diseases, it is not clear which cell to target with the normal gene. In cystic fibrosis, it is still not certain whether surface epithelial cells of the airway should be the target or whether transfection of submucosal gland epithelia should be the goal. In situations such as the prevention of restenosis by vascular smooth muscle cells of a coronary artery that has just been opened by percutaneous coronary angioplasty (PTCA) or in killing cancer cells the answer is obvious: target the site of disease. In immune deficiency diseases, hematologic stem cells might be the target. In hereditary bleeding disorders in which a circulating factor must be replaced or in AAT deficiency, there is a wide choice of cells that can be targeted for transfection (Fig. 5–3).

Ex vivo transfections are the answer in some settings. This was the technique used in the first trials of gene therapy for adenosine deaminase deficiency noted earlier. One approach to AAT deficiency has been to perform a partial hepatectomy (Fig. 5–4). The cultured hepatocytes are then transfected with the AAT gene. An antibiotic resistance gene is used to select transfected cells, which are then infused back into the portal venous system, repopulating the regenerating liver with hepatocytes expressing the normal AAT gene. Another ex vivo approach has been to take the patient's skin fibroblasts or muscle cells, transfect them in vitro, and reimplant them in skin or muscle or in the peritoneum or the intestinal omentum. In some instances, the transfected cells are embedded in a gel made of collagen that has angiogenic factors included in order to encourage vascularization of the embedded cells. These techniques have resulted in adequate levels of circulating AAT for weeks to months.

In vivo gene transfer into the liver and lung has been a major focus in AAT deficiency and in many hereditary diseases. In AAT deficiency, lung and liver cells have been selectively transfected, each generating significant local or circulating levels of AAT, at least for a short time. In each instance, selective targeting was achieved by using a tissue-specific route of gene delivery. For the lung, gene transfer has involved intratracheal instillation; for the liver, portal vein infusion has been used. Selective transfection of endothelial cells has been achieved by isolating a segment of blood vessel by balloon occlusion and introducing the vector into that segment, allowing time for the DNA to cross to endothelial cells before blood flow is re-established in the segment. This technique has been used to transfect a number of different genes in segments of coronary vessels that have undergone PTCA in order to

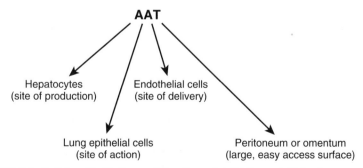

FIGURE 5–3. **Cell-Specific Delivery of the Normal AAT Gene.** AAT has been targeted to hepatocytes using ex vivo and in vivo techniques (see Fig. 5–4), to lungs by aerosol inhalation, to endothelial cells, and to the peritoneum and omentum by both ex vivo and in vivo approaches.

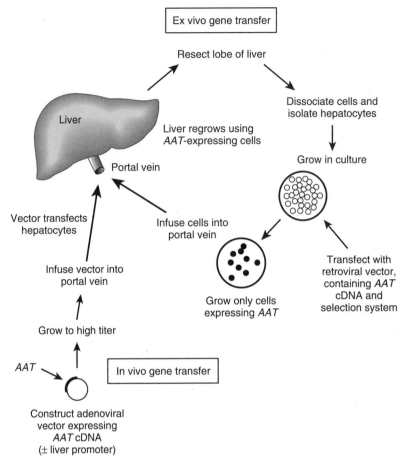

FIGURE 5–4. **Transfecting Hepatocytes with the AAT gene; Ex Vivo Versus In Vivo Approaches.** Ex vivo targeting of AAT involves performing a partial hepatectomy, transfecting cultured hepatocytes, selecting transfected cells, and reinfusing them in the regenerating liver. The liver regrows and incorporates AAT-producing cells. In vivo therapy has been performed using adenoviral AAT constructs, with the vectors being infused into the portal vein. Both methods have produced adequate circulating levels of AAT for some period of time.

prevent cells in that area from proliferating. Another approach to selective transfection of the brain has been to create an osmotic change in the blood-brain barrier prior to infusion with the gene of interest.

In vivo selective gene transfer continues to be an active area of investigation; one would like to kill only bad cells and fix only broken cells. Figure 5–5 illustrates a number of other methods that are being pursued to achieve tissue- or cell-specific gene transfer. They include targeting only dividing cells with retroviruses, adding gene-encoding ligands (e.g., antibodies, growth factors, cytokines, or SPA) that will bind to cell-specific receptors, and driving

Direct delivery

    Endothelium (intravenous or balloon occlusion)
    Hepatocytes (portal vein infusion)
    Lung epithelium (intratracheal or aerosol)
    Peritoneum (inject into, implant cells)
    Brain (inject into, alter blood-brain barrier)
    Tumors (inject into)

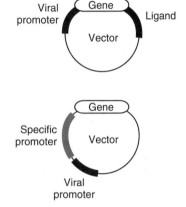

Ligand-receptor targeting

    Antibodies to cell-surface proteins
    Growth factors
    Cytokines
    Other ligands (e.g., SPA)

Cell-specific promoters

    von Willebrand's factor (endothelium)
    SP-C (type 2 cells)
    Albumin (liver)

FIGURE 5–5. **Strategies for Cell-Specific Gene Targeting.** Direct delivery of vectors has been accomplished in a variety of tissues. A variety of cell-specific ligands have been used to target cells, including SPA, which is taken up by an alveolar type 2 cell recycling pathway. In addition, genes have been expressed in specific tissues by insertion of a cell-specific promoter into the vector.

genes with promoters whose *trans*-acting factors are expressed only in the cell of interest, for example, using an SPC promoter to drive a gene that one wants to express only in type 2 cells.

## WHAT GENE TO USE?

It seems obvious that the gene to transfect is the normal form of the mutant gene. However, that might not always be the case. If one could correct the folding defect in cystic fibrosis or in AAT deficiency so that the protein could reach the apical cell surface in the case of *CFTR* or could be secreted in the case of AAT, one might not need to replace the mutant gene. In the case of cancer, there are a number of possible genes that might kill cancer cells without dealing with the causal defect in cancer, and in the case of preventing restenosis after PTCA, one is attempting to prevent the proliferation of vascular smooth muscle cells that limit the effectiveness of this procedure.

    Another decision that must be made is choosing which part of the selected DNA to insert into the vector. The coding region of a gene is not the only important portion of DNA. The 3′ part of the cDNA controls post-translational processing and the stability of the mRNA. One must make a decision as to how the transfected gene is to be regulated. In some instances, such as AAT, a strong constitutive promoter is all that is needed. In this setting, the gene remains "on" all the time. Even though AAT is an acute-phase reactant (i.e., it responds to acute stress), it is likely that constitutive expression is all that is needed. However, the highest levels of AAT that have yet been produced in transfection experiments have involved transfection of hepatocytes with AAT driven by a constitutive viral promoter as well as a liver-specific promoter.

When making decisions about the inserted DNA, it must also be ascertained whether it is important to know where the gene is expressed. If so, one must add some sort of reporter gene that will mark transfected cells.

## HOW LONG TO EXPRESS THE TRANSFECTED GENE?

For most acquired diseases, genes may need to be expressed for only short periods. When one wants to kill cancer or HIV-infected cells, a short period of gene transfer may be all that is needed. Conversely, most hereditary diseases require continuous expression of the missing or mutant gene. It is this need for prolonged expression that is the major impediment to effective gene therapy of diseases such as AAT deficiency and cystic fibrosis (see further on). At present, no system has been designed that provides high levels of gene product for long periods after a single transfection.

## HOW EFFICIENT DOES THE TRANSFECTION NEED TO BE?

The efficiency of a transfection is another important issue. Not all tumor cells need to be transfected with suicide genes; there is a bystander effect that kills adjacent untransfected cells (see Chapter 7). It has been determined that in monolayers of cystic fibrosis cells, only 20 to 40% of cells need to be transfected with normal *CFTR* for the ion transport defect to be corrected. In AAT deficiency, a serum level that is only 10 to 20% of normal achieves levels of AAT sufficient to prevent disease.

The efficiency of transfection is one of the most important limiting issues in gene transfer therapy, and there have been several approaches to improving efficiency, with many new methods on the way. Adding a positive charge to delivery systems increases the probability that endosomes will deliver the DNA to the nucleus, avoiding lysosomal degradation in the cytoplasmic compartment. Coinstillation or infusion of replication-deficient adenoviruses also increases endosomal activity at the cell surface, improving the delivery of DNA to the cell and avoiding lysosomal degradation. Other approaches are described in the following sections.

# How to Deliver the DNA

Delivery of the DNA is the major technical issue in gene therapy. Finding new ways to deliver genes with high efficiency and finding ways of expressing the genes for long periods with few side effects are the key issues facing gene therapists. There are two major methods for getting DNA into cells—viral vectors into which the foreign DNA has been inserted (Fig. 5–6) and DNA plasmids that are linked in some fashion to carriers that help the DNA get into the cell and avoid degradation in the cytoplasm. (Some of the methods for transfecting cells are illustrated in Figure 2–6.) Each method has advantages and disadvantages that are discussed further on. Although all the methods work, issues related to efficiency of transfection, cell targeting, amount of foreign DNA that can be carried, and side effects have combined to limit the effectiveness of gene therapy for most diseases and have led to the complete reassessment of the National Institutes of Health programs in gene therapy noted in the beginning of this chapter. Following is a brief review of several of the methods in use today.

## RETROVIRAL VECTORS

Retroviral vectors are RNA viruses that enter cells and are reverse transcribed into DNA. They are the vector that has been used most often in human trials to date. They have strong promoters that drive expression of inserted genes but relatively little space in which to insert foreign genes. Of course, the retroviral genome has been altered to remove the elements that are necessary for its independent replication (it is a replication-incompetent virus). Removing these elements provides room for insertion of the DNA to be transfected.

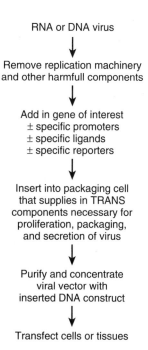

FIGURE 5–6. **Modifying Viral Vectors for Gene Transfer.** The first step in preparing viral vectors for gene transfection is to remove replication machinery so that the virus is unable to replicate on its own. Other potentially harmful portions of the viral genome, such as the immune-inducing portions of the adenovirus, are also removed. This provides room for insertion of the gene of interest, together with cell-specific promoters or ligands and reporter genes. The replication-incompetent viral vector is then grown in a packaging cell line that supplies the virus with the components necessary for replication. Once removed from the packaging cell, the virus is again unable to replicate. It is then purified and concentrated and transfected into the cell of interest.

These vectors can transfect dividing cells only, thus limiting their use in many adult tissues but improving their selectivity for cancer cells. Retroviruses insert into the genome of the transfected cell so that the vector and its accompanying DNA will be expressed in the transfected cell and passed on to all its daughter cells. Since the retroviral insertion occurs in a random fashion, there is no way to predict in what place and on which chromosome the virus is inserted. This random genomic insertion results in the theoretical concern that the retrovirus may activate an oncogene or may itself acquire replication capability.

To summarize, the advantage is genomic insertion and prolonged expression. The disadvantage is the limitation of transfection to proliferating cells and the limitation of the inserted DNA's size. The concern about subsequent mutagenesis and independent replication remains theoretical. There is active pursuit of new ways to target retroviral vectors more selectively.

## ADENOVIRAL VECTORS

Adenoviral vectors are DNA viruses that have strong promoters, can be easily grown in high titers, can accommodate relatively large pieces of inserted DNA, and can transfect nondividing cells. Some adenoviruses are trophic for airway epithelial cells, so they have been the vector of choice for introducing *CFTR* in cystic fibrosis patients. However, these vectors do not integrate into the host genome. Therefore, expression ceases when the transfected cell dies, since the gene is not passed on to daughter cells. This means continued expression requires repeated transfections and herein lies the problem with adenoviral vectors. They are immunogenetic, inducing a host immune response that results in T-cell–mediated killing of the very cells that express the transfected gene. The immune response is particularly vigorous on repeated transfections. Thus adenoviral vector gene expression persists for long periods in nude mice (with no immune response), for weeks to months after the first transfection in normal mice, and for days to weeks after succeeding transfections. The immune response has been so vigorous in some cystic fibrosis patients that they have experienced severe airway inflammation following repeated transfections. As with retroviral vectors, portions of the early adenoviral genes associated with viral replication (it is replication-incompetent) and adverse host responses have been deleted, which makes room for the inserted DNA.

To summarize, these are excellent vectors that can transfect nondividing cells, especially epithelial cells, but their inability to integrate into the genome requires repeated transfections that lead to severe immune responses. The future lies in eliminating additional parts of the adenoviral genome, which will, it is hoped, decrease its immunogenicity without sacrificing its advantages. Another approach has been to suppress the immune response to the transfected virus transiently (see Chapter 7).

## ADENO-ASSOCIATED VIRUS

Adeno-associated viruses (AAVs) belong to the parvovirus family. They integrate into the genome at a specific site on chromosome 19, so there are none of the concerns about random integration as with retroviruses. Genomic integration means prolonged expression, even in progeny of the transfected cells. AAVs are also nonimmunogenetic so that none of the adenoviral problems associated with immune inflammatory responses exist. However, the AAV genome is not large, limiting the size of the DNA that can be inserted to a few kilobases. In addition, there are technical problems with growing the virus and developing high titers for transfection.

In summary, these viruses have many good features, including a known site of genomic integration and lack of immunogenicity. A number of investigators are working on the technical limitations of the viruses, and there is hope that AAVs may be the vectors of the future.

## OTHER VIRAL VECTORS

Herpesvirus vectors have the advantage of being neurotrophic and can thus selectively target nondividing nerve cells. They also can accommodate large amounts of foreign DNA, up to 150 kb, and thus may be useful in combination with AAVs, which have a small capacity. Much work is being done to define the potential role of these and other viral vectors such as HIV and vaccinia.

## DNA-LIPID CONJUGATES

Liposomes are small spherical lipid vesicles that can be produced in vitro, stabilized, and then conjugated with DNA and various ligands that aid in targeting specific cells. Liposomes fuse with the cell membrane and enter the cell by endocytosis. The cationic liposomes and their conjugated DNA avoid intracellular degradation by remaining in the endosomal compartment (rather than in lysosomes) and deliver their DNA to the nucleus effectively. In general, they are preferentially targeted to cells of the reticuloendothelial system when given intravenously; thus, they are most effective when instilled directly into an organ such as the lung. They have no viral sequences and are nonimmunogenetic. They have low toxicity and thus can be given repeatedly, and they can transfect nondividing cells. They do not integrate into the host genome. Although their efficiency is less than that of viral systems, liposomes remain an important potential vector, especially for the lung, and new combinations with various ligands are being explored. Given the problems that have surfaced with adenoviral-induced inflammation in cystic fibrosis trials, liposome trials of *CFTR* transfer that are now under way have generated great interest.

## DNA RECEPTOR–LIGAND CONJUGATES

DNA can be directly conjugated with various ligands to target specific cells and when conjugated with positively charged material can avoid lysosomal degradation in the cell. This is a relatively new approach to gene transfer and is being studied intensely.

At present, human gene therapy is taking a breather. The focus is on solving problems with existing vectors and developing new ways of transfecting DNA in the most efficient fashion. New methods are evolving for cell-specific targeting of transfected DNA. Much work needs to be done to define stem cells in various tissues that might serve to populate tissues with gene-expressing cells throughout the life of the individual. Although there has been a momentary pause for reflection and experimentation, there is no question that human gene therapy will be an important part of the therapy of both acquired and hereditary human disease in the 21st century.

## SUGGESTED READING

### $\alpha_1$-Antitrypsin Deficiency

Carrell RW, Jeppsson J-O, Laurell C-B, et al: Structure and variation of human $\alpha_1$-antitrypsin. Nature 298:329–333, 1982.

Kalsheker KA: Molecular pathology of alpha 1-antitrypsin deficiency and its significance to clinical medicine. Q J Med 87:653–658, 1994.

Knoell DL, Wewers MD: Clinical implications of gene therapy for alpha$_1$-antitrypsin deficiency. Chest 107:535–545, 1995.

### Gene Therapy

Crystal RG: Transfer of genes to humans: Early lessons and obstacles to success. Science 270:404–409, 1995.

Kay MA, Graham F, Leland F, et al: Therapeutic serum concentrations of human alpha-1-antitrypsin after adenoviral-mediated gene transfer into mouse hepatocytes. Hepatology 21:815–819, 1995.

Marshall E: Special news report: Gene therapies growing pains. Science 269:1050–1055, 1995.

Moullier P, Bohl D, Cardoso J, et al: Long-term delivery of lysosomal enzyme by genetically-modified fibroblasts in dogs. Nat Med 1:353–358, 1995.

Verma IM, Somia N: Gene therapy—promises, problems and prospects. Nature 389:239–242, 1997.

Wilson JM: Adenoviruses as gene-delivery vehicles. N Engl J Med 334:1185–1187, 1996.

Yang Y, Trinchieri G, Wilson JM: Recombinant IL-12 prevents formation of blocking antibodies to recombinant adenovirus and allows repeated genetic treatment to mouse lung. Nat Med 1:890–893, 1995.

# Cystic Fibrosis: THE Genetic Disease

chromosomal jumping and walking •
positional cloning • protein structure-function
• post-translational processing •
recombinant proteins • cell-specific gene
targeting • splicing

Cystic fibrosis (CF) is the most common fatal autosomal recessive disease in Caucasians, with an incidence of 1 in 2500 live births. It results from the inheritance of two abnormal alleles on chromosome 7. Approximately 3.5% of Caucasians in the United States are heterozygous for CF, that is, they carry one abnormal allele. The defect that leads to the majority of CF symptoms, and ultimately to death, is in ion transport—both decreased outward flux of chloride and increased absorption of sodium. This results in the characteristic altered viscosity of exocrine gland secretions in the gut and lung that lead to pancreatic insufficiency and repeated pulmonary infections with progressive pulmonary insufficiency.

CF became the pulmonary disease most associated with the new science of molecular biology when the CF gene was identified in 1989. It was initially called the cystic fibrosis transmembrane conductance regulator (*CFTR*), and everything that has been learned about the protein since its discovery supports the wisdom of that name. The functions of *CFTR* are still being investigated, but it does act as a chloride ion channel as well as an adenosine triphosphate (ATP) channel, allowing efflux of both from the cell. In addition, it appears to regulate the functions of at least two other ion channels. The major CF mutations result in a chloride channel that does not respond to cAMP stimulation in a normal fashion and thus does not open to allow chloride flux from the cell in response to increased levels of cAMP. Chloride channel function is altered in CF, and in the most frequent CF mutations, CFTR fails to be transported to the apical cell surface.

The CF gene, which is on the long arm of chromosome 7, is large—250 kb with 27 exons; the mRNA is 6.2 kb, and the fully processed protein is 170 kd (see Fig. 1–7). It is highly glycosylated, has two membrane-spanning domains (each with six membrane-spanning segments), two ATP nucleotide-binding folds, and a regulatory region involved in cAMP-mediated phosphorylation (Fig. 6–1). The most common defect in CF, seen in 70% of patients, is a three-nucleotide, single-codon deletion that results in the loss of a single amino acid at position 508 (Δ508) located in the first nucleotide-binding fold. However, at least 500 other mutations have been described, most, in one way or another, leading to altered chloride channel function.

This chapter discusses the process of identifying a gene based on its chromosomal location (positional cloning), as well as techniques such as chromosome walking and jumping, which allow investigators to cover large portions of chromosomal DNA in the search for a disease-causing gene. However, finding the CF gene and characterizing its mutations was only the beginning. A major goal of research workers has been to define what the CF protein is, how it works, and how it is altered in disease. These studies provide an opportunity to discuss here how one predicts protein function from gene sequence, and the many mutations that have now been described in *CFTR* provide an opportunity to discuss the various ways in which an altered DNA sequence can influence the production of a protein.

One of the great surprises in defining the CF defect was the finding that the abnormal CFTR protein is not processed in a normal fashion after it is translated; in most cases it does not function normally because it is not transported to the apical cell surface. The defect in targeting CFTR to the right place provides an opportunity to discuss post-translational regulation of proteins, that is, the processing of proteins after they have left the ribosome.

Treatment of CF in the pre–molecular biology era had a profound effect on survival and the quality of life. Treatment of infection, improved nutrition, and improved bronchial drainage have increased the median age of survival of these patients into the mid-30s. Despite the tremendous excitment generated by the discovery of the CF gene and by attempts at gene therapy, to date modern molecular biology has added little of substance to the treatment

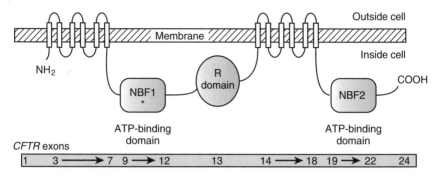

500 different cystic fibrosis mutations spread throughout gene

*$^{2}/_{3}$ of mutations at codon 508 in exon 10

Membrane-spanning domains
viewed from above

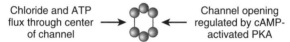

Chloride and ATP
flux through center → ← Channel opening
of channel regulated by cAMP-
activated PKA

FIGURE 6–1. **Deduced Protein Structure of CFTR.** *CFTR* has 12 membrane-spanning domains, two nucleotide-binding folds *(NBF1* and *NBF2)*, a regulatory domain *(R)*, and an amino *(NH$_2$)* terminus and a carboxyl *(COOH)* terminus. The membrane-spanning segments form a channel, viewed from the surface of the cell membrane, through which chloride and adenosine triphosphate *(ATP)* flow. This flux is regulated by cAMP activation of protein kinase A *(PKA)*. Depicted beneath are the exons, coding for each portion of *CFTR.* Although mutations have been described in virtually every exon, the most common mutation is a deletion of codon 508 in exon 10. This amino acid lies in NBF1 (° in *NBF1).* (See text for description of major types of *CFTR* mutations and their physiologic consequences.) The bottom of the figure shows a view of *CFTR* from the top of a membrane, illustrating its channel structure.

of CF, other than hope, with one exception. This exception provides an opportunity to discuss recombinant or genetically engineered proteins, in this case human DNase I (rhDNase).

Recent discoveries about CF have proved among the most exciting applications of molecular biology to human disease. The finding of the CF gene, definition of its mutations, analysis of the effect of altered structure on protein function, attempts to target expression of the normal CF gene to specific cells and tissues, and the emergence of tests for the prenatal diagnosis of CF have all occurred within the last several years. They have had profound effects on science and medicine and have generated hope for CF patients and their families. They have also provided an important boost for advocates of basic science research.

## Finding the Cystic Fibrosis Gene: Jumping and Walking to *CFTR*

The story of how the CF gene was found produced headlines in the lay and scientific press in the late 1980s, in part because of the importance of the disease, in part because of the new concepts and new methods that were being worked out that would establish a strategy for finding other genes whose functions were not known, and in part because of the fame and fortune that would be heaped on the "winner of the race." In 1988, *Science* reviewed the progress in an article entitled "The Race for the Cystic Fibrosis Gene" with the following quote, "This is not your average ego-driven science. This is nasty." However, as is increasingly the case with molecular biologic research, it took a large collaborative group and considerable sharing of information to make the discovery. Three articles describing the CF gene and declaring that the search had ended were published in *Science* in 1989. They included a total of 25 authors from five institutions using consortium-derived genetic material for analysis, a variety of biochemical and molecular techniques, and funding from myriad public and private agencies. In addition, the group worked from a background of genetic markers spanning chromosome 7 that had been described previously by numerous investigators.

The search for the CF gene involved new concepts and resulted in the development of a number of novel methods. Until this time, genes had been found by functional cloning. In this strategy, a disease was described, a protein was implicated in its pathogenesis, the protein was sequenced, and the gene was found by probing a cDNA library with oligonucleotides deduced from the protein sequence. However, for the vast majority of genetic diseases, this strategy has not been useful because the mutant protein and its function usually are not known. The approach taken for CF involved a technique called positional cloning or reverse genetics. In this strategy, data from a large number of CF families with several generations of genetic information are collected and the relation between inheritance of a number of polymorphic genetic markers (see Chapter 3) and the disease is explored. The suspect gene is localized to a region or position on a chromosome and then it is identified, cloned, and sequenced; its function is determined; and the mutations responsible for the disease are defined. This is hard work, which, in the case of CF, took many investigator hours, since much of the human genome was still not mapped at the time the studies were carried out. The more the human genome is mapped, the easier the process will be for future genes (see Chapter 10).

The localization process involved finer and finer definition of the gene's site (Fig. 6–2). The first steps in locating the CF gene used techniques described in Chapter 3. Linkage analysis compares the inheritance of polymorphic gene markers (i.e., markers that are in different forms on maternal and paternal alleles) to inheritance of disease in large family cohorts; the closer a marker and a disease gene, the more likely they are to be coinherited.

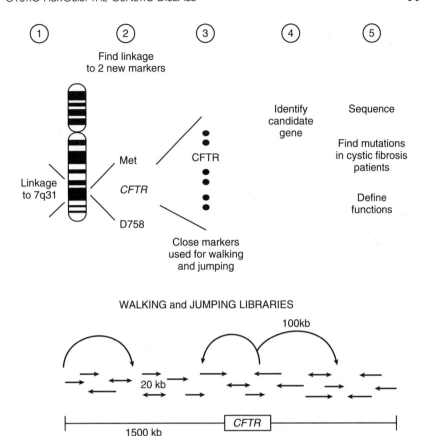

FIGURE 6–2. **The Positional Cloning Approach to Identifying *CFTR*.** Initially, cystic fibrosis (CF) was linked to a marker that proved to be on the long arm of chromosome 7 *(1)*. New linkage markers were discovered that bracketed the putative CF gene *(2)*, and then additional markers were found that closed in on the gene, narrowing the search to an area that spanned 1 to 2 centimorgans on chromosome 7 *(3)*. These markers were then used as starting points for walking down the chromosome or jumping large distances across the chromosome. Not all walking proceeded in the same direction. This approach, described in the text, was combined with developing criteria for a candidate gene *(4)* (see Table 6–1). The *CFTR* was eventually identified in a cDNA library made from the sweat glands of a patient with CF. Once identified, the gene can be sequenced, mutations in CF patients defined, and protein functions determined.

Early studies of CF families linked the disease to an anonymous marker (a marker with no known function) whose chromosomal location was not initially known. Subsequent studies focused on the long arm of chromosome 7, and a series of studies from different laboratories all using similar techniques placed the CF gene between two markers 1 million to 2 million base pairs (1 to 2 centimorgans) apart at chromosome 7q31.2–3.

Once the general location of the CF gene was defined, investigators needed a new strategy to find the CF gene itself because further linkage analysis could not narrow gene-to-marker distances of less than approximately 1 million base pairs. This required new markers that covered the area between the flanking markers, new methods to move up or down the chromosome toward the putative CF site, and new ideas for identifying candidate genes. A number of additional anonymous markers were described that covered the region. The distance between the flanking markers was covered by walking or jumping down the chromosome while looking for the gene (see Fig. 6–2). This required making genomic DNA walking and jumping libraries. The 1.5 million base pair region was cut into small or very large pieces with either common or rare cutter restriction endonucleases. The smaller pieces were cloned into cosmid vectors as described in Chapter 2. This DNA library covered the whole area of interest in pieces of DNA that were 10 kb. The investigators could begin with a probe for one of the previously described markers and use that probe to find the next overlapping piece of DNA. That piece was then sequenced or used as a probe to find the next overlapping piece, and so on, moving slowly toward the CF gene. This method could be used to walk in either direction. The process was extremely laborious, and often there were pieces of DNA that could not be cloned for technical reasons, which interrupted the walk. To overcome these problems, jumping libraries were invented. This involved taking big pieces of DNA (100 kb) and circularizing them so that the ends met at a ligation site. One could then clone the overlapping ends of large circular pieces of DNA, in essense jumping over the large piece of DNA that would have taken many probes and much time to walk through. The combination of the two approaches moved investigators closer to the putative CF site, but how did they know when they had arrived and how did they identify the candidate gene?

This again required new ideas (Table 6–1). It is known that at the 5′ end of most mammalian genes, there is a region that is rich in cytosines and guanines. These regions, called CpG islands (see also Chapter 7), often signal the start of a new gene, and they were used to identify genes within the jumping and walking libraries. A second way to determine when one has reached an important gene is to see if the DNA sequence is conserved across species. Most important genes are present in mammalian as well as invertebrate species. (Such conservation of genes was described in Chapters

TABLE 6–1
*Identifying Candidate Genes*

| |
|---|
| CpG islands mark the 5′ end of most genes |
| Important genes are conserved across species |
| Is the DNA expressed in the appropriate tissues? |
| Are there mutations in the DNA of patients? |
| Does the function of the protein relate to the disease? |

2 and 3 and is discussed further in Chapter 8.) A third method was to see if the candidate gene is expressed in appropriate tissues; for CF, it was clear that the important tissues were at least lung, sweat glands, and intestine. If the mRNA was not expressed on Northern blots of these tissues, it was not likely to be the CF gene. It then had to be shown that the gene was present in CF patients and that CF patients had some mutation in the gene. A piece of one candidate gene was identified this way, and a probe from that piece of DNA was used to screen a cDNA library, that is, a DNA library that coded only for mRNA without all the intronic and other DNA junk that is present in genomic DNA libraries. This probe identified the *CFTR*, which was cloned and sequenced and in the majority of CF patients displayed the Δ508 single codon mutation. Further, as will be discussed later, the *CFTR* was shown to be a chloride channel whose physiology was altered in a fashion compatible with differences in chloride flux that had been observed in epithelial cells of CF patients. Once the gene and the predominant mutation were found, exploration of its physiology, creation of animal models, gene therapy, genetic testing, and much more were possible and, in addition, a new approach to finding genes that cause human disease—positional cloning—had been described. This method has subsequently been used to find a number of other disease-causing genes.

## Correlating DNA Sequence with Protein Function

How does one determine the function of a gene from its DNA sequence? Indeed, how was it determined that *CFTR* was a chloride channel and had membrane-spanning domains and an ATP-binding pocket? Today, the answer is simple. One goes to the computer, links up to a gene data bank or one of a number of special computer programs, enters the DNA sequence of the gene, and asks the computer questions. The question can be, What is the deduced protein sequence, that is, the sequence of amino acids encoded by the gene's open reading frame? Are there any genes or proteins like this one in the computer and what do they do? Are there parts of this gene that are like any other gene? From the predicted amino acid sequence, can one predict the secondary structure of this protein? One can even ask if there is a homologous gene that has been described and whose function has been determined in a different animal species, bacteria, or yeast? Thus, many answers about structure and function now come from a comfortable chair and a computer. Most journals require assurance that information about the sequence of new genes be entered in universally available data banks before they agree to publish an article describing a new gene.

On occasion, a gene is found that is unlike anything ever seen before. This is both a scientist's dream and a potential nightmare. The dream is to get there first; the nightmare is the possibility that one cannot determine the function of the gene discovered. Most often, genes are found because one is investigating a function. However, sometimes one finds a gene for which the data banks do not help and there is not a clue. Gene knockouts may help, but if the gene is really important, knockouts are either embryonic lethals (the embryo dies in utero) or there is so much redundancy built into the biologic system that there is no knockout phenotype (see Chapter 4).

However, to prove that CFTR really transported chloride, investigators had to transfect the *CFTR* cDNA into a cell that did not contain a cAMP-activated chloride channel and show that chloride flux changed in the presence of the transfected cDNA and that it was cAMP-sensitive. To demonstrate what each part of the protein does, one has to mutate the cDNA and determine how that mutation affects function or regulation of the protein. Once this has been carried out for one gene, homologous genes can be expected to function in the same fashion.

It has been known for some time that abnormal cAMP-mediated chloride transport was not the only defect in CF. Airway epithelial sodium secretion is increased, as is calcium-mediated chloride channel activity. The function of another type of chloride channel (the outward-rectifying chloride channel) is also impaired in CF. The cloning of *CFTR* and the availability of a number of CF and normal epithelial cell lines have allowed investigators to examine ion transport via other channels in CF cells and then to test the effect of correcting the ion transport defects by transfecting CF cells with normal *CFTR*. These studies have shown that CFTR not only transports chloride on its own but also regulates ion transport by other channels (Fig. 6–3). CFTR regulates the outward-rectifying chloride channel by transporting ATP outside the cells, and this ATP then activates the outward-rectifying chloride channel via a purinergic-type receptor on the same epithelial cells. In CF, ATP transport through CFTR is impaired, and therefore the outward-rectifying chloride channel does not function normally. Transfecting CF cells with normal *CFTR* also corrects both increased sodium reabsorption and calcium-mediated chloride transport, suggesting that CFTR also regulates these ion channels. Since the cAMP-sensitive sodium-absorbing channel has been cloned, the interaction between normal *CFTR* and the sodium channel can be studied and the defect in sodium transport in CF defined. Using cells that normally express neither channel, investigators have cotransfected CFTR and sodium channels and found that cAMP opens *CFTR*, allowing chloride efflux while also decreasing sodium influx. The mutant CFTR results in increased basal sodium influx with additional sodium influx in response to cAMP. Thus, CFTR normally suppresses activity of the sodium-resorbing channel via cAMP, but mutant *CFTR* fails to regulate the sodium channel cAMP response. The discussion of translational processing of proteins also suggests that CFTR regulates Golgi compartment pH, affecting protein sialylation in that compartment. Thus, CFTR serves multiple regulatory functions in addition to its own critical role as a chloride transporter.

The high frequency of mutations in this critical ion transporter and ion

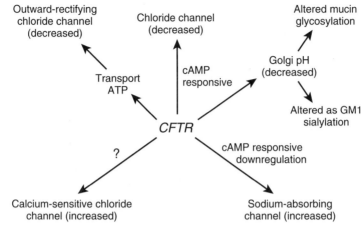

FIGURE 6–3. **CFTR Functions.** CFTR has been found to have a number of functions in addition to acting as a chloride channel. Under normal circumstances, CFTR allows chloride flux in response to cAMP. CFTR has also been shown to transport ATP, which, in turn, regulates an outward-rectifying chloride channel. Whether CFTR also regulates a calcium-sensitive chloride channel is not clear. This channel increases activity in CF versus the decrease in function of the other two channels. CFTR has recently been shown to influence the function of a sodium-absorbing channel that is cAMP-responsive, although the mechanism is not clear. Finally, CFTR appears to affect the pH of the Golgi apparatus by an unclear mechanism, altering glycosylation and sialylation of mucin and other glycoproteins and glycolipids.

transport regulator that has persisted for generations raises the issue of why such a potentially lethal mutation has remained in our gene pool. Geneticists have argued for years that some survival advantage must be conferred to heterozygotes (carriers) of CF by the *CFTR* mutation. As an example, sickle cell heterozygotes are protected against malaria. In the case of CF, a recent study of *CFTR* gene knockout mice has shown that CF mutations protect against the secretory diarrhea induced by cholera toxin during infection with *Vibrio cholerae*. Cholera induces severe diarrhea and death by elevating colonic epithelial cell cAMP, with resulting massive chloride and fluid secretion. It has long been suspected that CF might protect against the effects of cholera because intestinal epithelial cells expressing mutant *CFTR* would not respond to increased levels of cAMP with chloride flux. This proved to be the case in *CFTR* knockout mice. When given cholera toxin, homozygotes (with no intestinal CFTR) had 25% of the intestinal fluid secretion of normal mice, whereas heterozygotes (with 50% of normal CFTR protein) had 50% less. This demonstrates that CF does protect against the diarrhea of cholera and may provide CF patients with a selective survival advantage, at least in areas where cholera is endemic, thus providing one explanation for the high incidence of CF carriers.

## *CFTR* Mutations: What Kind and What Do They Mean?

By now more than 500 mutations have been described in *CFTR*. Sixty-five to 70% of these mutations result in deletion of the phenylalanine, which lies in an ATP-binding fold at codon 508 (see Fig. 6–1). The frequency of this mutation varies among populations so that in the south of Europe the Δ508 deletion occurs in only 20% of CF cases, whereas in Denmark it occurs in more than 90% of CF cases. In Israel, a missense mutation (a mutation that changes but does not delete an amino acid) occurs in 60% of Ashkenazi Jews with CF, but appears in only 2% of all CF patients that have been studied worldwide. This type of variability in *CFTR* mutations is of interest to population geneticists who can use them to trace the origins of *CFTR* mutations.

All DNA mutations are not equal. Of the 500 mutations described to date, not all are associated with disease. Some completely prevent production of CFTR; others have no effect at all on CFTR protein production or function. Since so many mutations have been described in CF patients, this chapter discusses the types of DNA mutations that can occur and their consequences.

The various mutations described in CF also provide important insights into CFTR function. The general types of gene mutations are illustrated and discussed in Chapter 3. Four general types of mutations have been described in CF. Although the vast majority of mutations result in defective processing of CFTR, other mutations, although rare, provide insights into CFTR function. Some mutations are null mutations, that is, they result in *little or no CFTR protein.* These usually occur because a nonsense mutation, a frameshift mutation, or a splice site mutation (see further on) results in a premature stop codon that terminates translation of the protein. This usually results in severe disease because no CFTR protein is produced. The most common types of CF mutations result in *defective processing of* CFTR (see next section) so that it does not reach the cell surface where it performs its functions. These are usually codon deletions or point mutations that occur in the nuclear binding folds and presumably alter protein conformation or folding. The third type of mutation occurs as a result of point mutations in the nuclear binding fold and results in *defective regulation of* CFTR that has been processed normally so that it reaches the cell surface. Point mutations have been described in the transmembrane portions of CFTR, the presumed chloride channels. These defects result in *altered properties of the ion channel* and impaired ion flow, but membrane location of the CFTR and its regulation are normal. Finally, there are mutations that do not appear to affect the function of CFTR or result in a clinical phenotype.

For a number of years, investigators have attempted to correlate *CFTR* mutations with clinical manifestations of disease. Before the CF gene was identified, investigators had predicted a relation between the severity of pancreatic disease and the type of mutation. To a degree, this has proved to be the case, but studies to date have failed to provide a clear-cut link between specific mutations and clinical disease except for the pancreatic insufficiency. Null mutations and mutations that affect processing, such as Δ 508, produce severe pancreatic insufficiency. Mutations that affect the channel itself but do not affect *CFTR* processing or regulation tend to have mild pancreatic insufficiency. To confuse the picture, however, some patients with classic Δ508 mutations have no phenotype other than sterility because of the absence of the vas deferens.

## A New Mutation Associated with Normal Sweat Chloride Concentrations: RNA Splicing Problems

In most instances, mutations that occur in introns do not affect protein structure or function, since introns are eliminated in the processing of RNA and do not participate in protein synthesis. This is true except for the highly conserved intron sequences that mark the splice sites for removal of introns during the nuclear processing of pre-mRNA to mRNA. The key to removing introns lies in the sequences at intron-exon boundaries. At the 5′ end of the intron, a GT sequence in DNA marks a splice site (the donor site) and at the 3′ end of the intron, an AG sequence identifies the other intron-exon boundary (the acceptor site). The splicesome is a complex of small nuclear RNAs and other nuclear proteins (called heterogeneous RNA or hnRNA) that recognize specific sequences at intron-exon junctions of pre-mRNA and regulate the excision of introns. The 5′ end is first cleaved and bends over toward the 3′ end, forming a circular structure. The 3′ end is then cleaved and the intron is removed to be degraded in the nucleus, whereas the ends of the exons are joined to one another. The signal nucleotides at either end of the intron regulate the site of splicing (Fig. 6–4).

Some single gene transcripts can be spliced in different ways, giving rise to more than one mRNA and occasionally more than one protein. There can be two forms of the same protein or two different proteins that arise from a single gene. The mechanisms of this process, called alternative splicing, are not completely worked out. However, it appears that different proteins expressed in different cells can act in *trans* to influence what is spliced in or out by skipping or including various exons. Acting in *trans*, as in the discussion of transcriptional gene regulation in Chapter 8, means that a cell makes a protein that binds to DNA and influences the processing of that DNA. Thus, proteins that block or provide access to splice sites may provide a mechanism for cell-specific alternative splicing. Examples include the α-tropomyosin gene, which has 14 exons that are alternatively spliced to form different types of myosin in skeletal muscle, smooth muscle, and fibroblasts; fibronectin, which has 50 exons that are alternatively spliced to form circulating, mem-

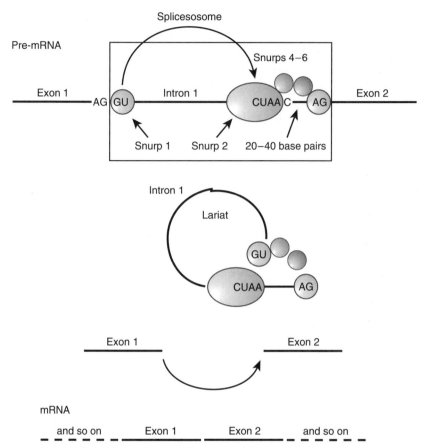

FIGURE 6–4. **Splicing Out Introns to Form mRNA.** Intron-exon boundaries are marked by a 5' intronic GT in DNA or GU in RNA (the donor site) and an AG at the 3' end (the acceptor site). As discussed in the text, a complex of small nuclear particles (snurps) assembles at the 5' end of the intron, which is cleaved and bent to form a lariat-shaped structure, connecting at a crucial A in the snurp 2 complex. Following cleavage at the AG site, the intron is degraded and the exons are joined.

brane-bound, and matrix-associated fibronectins; and the calcitonin-CGRP gene, which is alternatively spliced to produce calcitonin in the thyroid and CGRP in the brain. At a more basic level, alternative splicing in *Drosophila* controls the expression of male versus female sex.

When a mutation occurs at either of the key GT or AG boundary nucleotides, introns are not cut out in a normal fashion and splicing variants may lead to abnormal mRNA and protein. Recently, such a mutation was reported in a group of CF patients (Fig. 6–5). This variation appears to occur, for as yet unexplained reasons, in individuals with less severe lung disease who have normal sweat chloride concentrations. The mutation appears to account for the majority of individuals with signs and symptoms of CF but

Intron mutation in cystic fibrosis patients with normal sweat chlorides

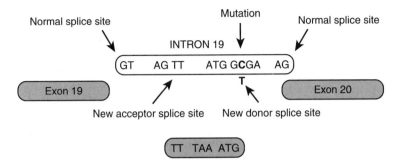

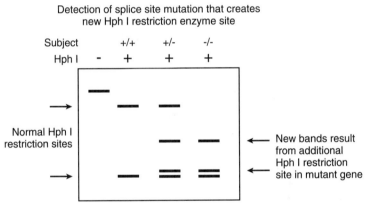

FIGURE 6–5. **A CF Mutation with Normal Sweat Chloride Concentrations: An Altered Splice Site.** A DNA mutation of a C to a T (or U in RNA) in intron 19 of the *CFTR* introduces a new premature acceptor splice site *(arrow)*. A cryptic (previously unused) donor splice site *(arrow)* is activated, creating two splicing events in the intron. This results in a piece of the intron (starting with *TT* and ending with *ATG*) being connected to exons 19 and 20. The newly included piece contains within it a stop codon *(TAA)* that prematurely terminates translation of the CFTR protein. This inclusion also creates a new internal Hph I restriction enzyme cutting site, resulting in a diagnostic restriction fragment length polymorphism (RFLP).

normal sweat chloride concentrations and thus provides a means of making a specific diagnosis in these previously difficult to diagnose patients.

The mutation is within an intron producing a C to T DNA change (or C to U in RNA), resulting in a GT sequence that becomes a new splice donor site within intron 19. The new splice site results in the activation of a cryptic (previously unused) acceptor splice site further upstream toward the 5′ end of intron 19. The result is two splicing events in intron 19, with the joining of an 84–base pair segment of intron 19 to exons 19 and 20 (see Fig. 6–5).

The included segment of intron contains an in-frame stop codon that serves to end CFTR protein synthesis before exon 20, which codes for the ATP-binding pocket at the carboxyl terminus of the protein. The C to T mutation also creates a new restriction enzyme cutting site for the endonuclease Hhp I which recognizes the sequence GGTGT. This results in a restriction fragment length polymorphism for the mutation illustrated in Figure 6–5, thus providing a simple means of diagnosing the mutation. It turns out that a small amount of normal *CFTR* is present in persons who have this mutation, presumably resulting in sufficient normal CFTR protein to produce normal sweat chloride concentrations and relatively mild pancreatic and respiratory disease. The report of this mutation, together with a simple method of diagnosis, means that the definition of CF can now be extended in a reliable fashion to patients who have suppurative pulmonary disease and normal sweat chloride concentrations.

## What Is the Problem with Δ508 *CFTR*?: Post-translational Processing of Proteins

One of the great surprises of the early studies of the *CFTR* gene was the observation that mutant CFTR might not be functional because it does not reach the apical cell membrane where it normally functions. Indeed, the most common form of CF mutation, Δ508, results in CFTR remaining in the endoplasmic reticulum (ER) and not appearing on the apical cell surface of human CF cells (see Fig. 6–6). If mutant CFTR can be induced to reach the cell surface, its function is only slightly impaired. Understanding the reason for this surprising result requires a brief discussion of post-translational regulation of gene expression, that is, an understanding of how a protein is fully processed and is sent to its site of function after it is initially produced on cytoplasmic ribosomes. Just as RNA is processed after it has been transcribed in order to serve its function (post-transcriptional processing), proteins are processed after they have been translated in order to serve their function (post-translational processing).

As was discussed in Chapter 1, the cell nucleus is the site of DNA and RNA synthesis, whereas the cytoplasm is the site of protein and lipid synthesis and processing. The cytoplasm consists of the cytosol and a number of specialized organelles. The largest of these organelles, the ER, lies adjacent to the nucleus; it is where ribosomes attach and where noncytoplasmic protein synthesis, as well as lipid synthesis, occurs. In addition, glycosylation of proteins begins here, as does the folding of proteins as they assume their three-dimensional structure (Fig. 6–7; see also Chapter 5).

Since unfolded proteins are able to fold spontaneously in a test tube, it had long been assumed that all the information required for protein folding was contained in the charge and hydrophobicity of the amino acids that make up the protein. Recently, a large class of proteins called chaperones has been

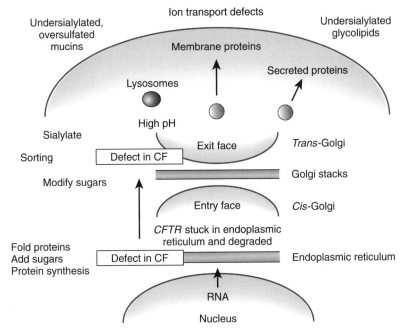

FIGURE 6–6. **CFTR from Gene to Protein.** Processing of the *CFTR* DNA and defects found in Δ508 mutation. (See text for explanation.)

discovered that function to induce protein folding and stabilize tertiary protein structure. Studies have shown that a chaperone, HS-70, associates with CFTR in the ER and then dissociates from normal CFTR as it moves to the Golgi apparatus. In contrast, HS-70 does not dissociate from mutant CFTR, and the complex remains in the ER to be degraded. For some reason, when folding cannot occur, the chaperone does not dissociate from the protein, the unfolded protein does not move to the next processing compartment, and the protein is degraded.

The Golgi apparatus serves as a central clearing house, where proteins and lipids from the ER are accepted, modified, and then routed to other destinations or kept to perform specific functions in the ER or Golgi apparatus. The fate of these proteins is guided in large part by signals incorporated into their peptide structure. The Golgi apparatus is also a major site of carbohydrate synthesis. These carbohydrates are most often side chains attached to the proteins that have been made in the ER. Each Golgi apparatus, which is actually a series of tubules, has an ER side, the *cis* or entry face, and a non-ER side, the *trans* or exit face. Proteins that enter the Golgi on the *cis* side can either move to the *trans* network of the Golgi apparatus or return to the ER. Proteins that exit the *trans* Golgi apparatus move to lysosomes, to the cell surface, or to secretory vesicles. This processing system is important not only in targeting proteins and lipids to their proper destina-

CFTR from gene to protein
(and defect in Δ508 mutation)

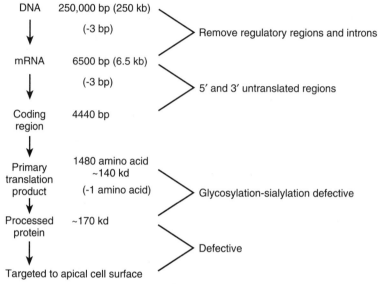

FIGURE 6–7. **Post-Translational Processing of *CFTR;* The Problem with Δ508.** Under normal circumstances, proteins that are to be transported from the cell are synthesized in the endoplasmic reticulum, sugars begin to be added, and folding of the proteins occurs. These proteins shuttle to the *cis,* or entry, Golgi stacks, where sugars are modified; some proteins return to the endoplasmic reticulum; and others move through the Golgi stacks to the *trans* Golgi apparatus, where sorting to final destination occurs and terminal glycosylation and sialylation take place. Proteins then move to the cell surface and are secreted or enter lysosomal compartments for degradation or recycling. In CF, the most prevalent mutation (Δ508) is associated with defective folding so that the CFTR never leaves the endoplasmic reticulum. A second abnormality appears to occur in the *trans* Golgi apparatus, where acidification of the Golgi apparatus is defective and sialylation of mucin and glycolipids is altered.

tions but also in modifying them by the addition or rearrangement of carbohydrates so that they can assume their final structure and function.

The *trans* Golgi apparatus normally has a low pH, and this acidic environment plays an important role in the activity of the enzymes that add carbohydrates to proteins and lipids in the Golgi apparatus. Further, it appears that the acidity of the *trans* Golgi vesicles is regulated by Golgi apparatus chloride channels. Golgi apparatus chloride transport, perhaps regulated directly by CFTR or another channel that is regulated by CFTR, is defective in cells transfected with the Δ508 *CFTR* and is corrected by transfection with normal *CFTR.*

As a result of the abnormal pH of the *trans* Golgi apparatus, glycosylation of other cell surface and secreted proteins and lipids is also affected in CF (see Fig. 6–6). It has long been known that the airway secretions of CF patients are not only thick and viscid but also undersialylated and oversulfated. Sialic acid is one of the last sugar residues added to glycoproteins and glycolipids in the *trans* Golgi apparatus, and the process of sialylation and sulfation are competitive. It would appear that if sialic acid is not added in mutant *CFTR* epithelial cells, sulfate is added instead. When cells making undersialylated glycoproteins are transfected with wild-type *CFTR*, the defect in sialylation is corrected.

Does altered protein or lipid sialylation have any biologic consequences in CF? Recent studies suggest that these changes in Golgi apparatus function may be responsible for the *Pseudomonas* colonization and infections that plague CF patients. Gangliosides are complex combinations of lipid with sugar side chains that contain one or more terminal sialic acid residues. One of these gangliosides, $GM_1$, acts as a cell surface receptor for the toxin that causes diarrhea in cholera. The gram-negative bacterium *Pseudomonas aeruginosa* can recognize the terminal sugars in nonsialylated or asialo-$GM_1$. CF epithelial cells with $\Delta508$ express *asialo*-$GM_1$, and bind *Pseudomonas* organisms, whereas normal epithelial cells or CF cells transfected with wild-type *CFTR* express *sialylated* $GM_1$ and bind *Pseudomonas* with much lower affinity. The same is true for *Staphylococcus aureus*. Antibodies to asialo-$GM_1$ block binding of *Pseudomonas*. Thus, the altered *trans* Golgi apparatus pH and resultant undersialylation of proteins and lipids in the Golgi apparatus may explain the propensity for *Pseudomonas* and staphyloccocal infection in CF patients. If investigators can correct the *trans* Golgi apparatus pH defect, they may, by increasing glycolipid sialylation, prevent $GM_1$ from binding organisms such as *P. aeruginosa* and *S. aureus*.

In retrospect, there was a clue to the *CFTR* defect and its treatment in early studies of CFTR that demonstrated that CFTR was a chloride channel. These experiments involved transfection of *CFTR* into the frog oocyte. The oocyte is a favorite model for ion transport scientists, because it is a large, simple cell that can be immobilized and punctured to study intracellular ion concentrations and ion fluxes. When the *CFTR* gene was first cloned, it was expressed in frog oocytes, and it induced a chloride channel on the cell surface. The $\Delta508$ mutant *CFTR* also appeared at the oocyte cell surface but did not open normally to allow chloride flux in the presence of cAMP. Subsequent studies of CFTR in mammalian cells, discussed earlier, showed that normal or wild-type CFTR appeared at the cell surface but that mutant CFTR did not. Since oocytes are routinely cultured at 30 to 32°C, investigators lowered the temperature of mammalian cells (usually kept at 37°C) transfected with mutant *CFTR* and the protein appeared at the cell surface and functioned in a relatively normal fashion. The explanation for this temperature-dependent movement in $\Delta508$ CFTR to the cell surface probably lies in the effect that temperature has on protein folding.

Two genetically determined pulmonary diseases, CF and $\alpha_1$-antitrypsin deficiency (see Chapter 5), are associated with defects in protein folding. Advances in the field of molecular chaperones and in the biophysics of protein folding are likely to provide new tools for understanding, and possibly treating, these two pulmonary diseases. Should release of unfolded proteins or correction of folding defects become possible, CF may ultimately be treated without the need for *CFTR* gene therapy.

## Animal Models of Cystic Fibrosis: Cell-Specific Targeting of Genes

Once the CF gene was identified and cloned, investigators quickly set to work on producing *CFTR* knockout mice using the techniques described in Chapter 4. The advantages of having an animal model of the human disease are obvious, particularly when it comes to designing drugs that might overcome the defect in chloride flux, the post-translational defect in CFTR, and the respiratory tract infections that lead to death in most patients. Three research groups published *CFTR* knockout animal model results within a month of one another in 1992. As one might predict, none of the models exactly reproduced the human disease. All models displayed abnormal epithelial cell chloride conductance similar to that seen in humans and thus proved that there is no backup system for the CFTR. There was no genetic redundancy for *CFTR*, that is, no gene coding for another channel took over the functions of *CFTR*.

Redundancy has been the case in many knockout mice, especially in studies of the role of regulators of gene expression during development. As an example, retinoic acid receptors (RARs) are important modulators of the response to retinoic acid and are thought to be involved in the structural organization of many developing tissues, including the lung. Knocking out either RAR receptor, RARα or β$_2$, both of which are expressed in the developing lung, produces no recognizable phenotype and no apparent alteration in lung development. However, when RARα knockout mice were bred with RARβ$_2$ knockout mice, the resulting double knockout offspring express neither receptor, and all double knockouts displayed agenesis or hyoplasia of the lungs. Thus RARα and RARβ$_2$ overlap in their functions during lung development; when one is absent, the other provides a backup function. When both are absent, no lung forms. Thus, the RAR system is redundant, at least for lung development. As discussed in Chapter 4, creating a "knockin" mouse that replaces one RAR receptor with another, with the second receptor expressed in the same cells and at the same time as the first receptor, would tell us whether RARα serves exactly the same functions as RARβ$_2$.

Two of the *CFTR* knockouts, using a targeted insertion that eliminated part of the normal *CFTR*, produced mice that died of intestinal obstruction and perforation within the first month of life. The mutation used to produce the *CFTR* knockout involved insertion of a stop codon in exon 10 that resulted in a truncated gene product similar to that seen in some CF patients with Δ508 mutation. Although the lesions were similar to the human intestinal disease associated with CF, they were so severe that the animals never lived to acquire respiratory disease.

All that work making a *CFTR* knockout and yet no animal model of human respiratory disease. As always with molecular biology, it took only bright minds employing the tricks of molecular biology to solve the problem. The solution was to prevent the gastrointestinal disease, allowing the mice to live long enough for the pulmonary disease to evolve so that it could be studied. The strategy was to create a transgenic knockout mouse in which the transgene replaced the knocked-out gene, but only in the gastrointestinal tract. The trick was to put a gastrointestinal tract cell–specific promoter in front of the normal *CFTR* and make transgenic mice that were heterozygous for *CFTR*. These mice, which were *CFTR* +/− were then mated with other heterozygotes not expressing the transgene. Some offspring were CFTR −/− everywhere except in the gastrointestinal tract, where wild-type *CFTR* was fully expressed. These mice are now being followed for the development of respiratory disease. The concept of tissue- and cell-specific gene regulation is discussed in Chapter 8.

The third group targeted a premature stop codon without otherwise altering the *CFTR* and produced a mouse with no phenotype, that is, no recognizable disease. These animals produced small amounts of normal *CFTR* (and thus had a "leaky" knockout). When kept in a germ-free environment, they did not develop overt disease and had perfectly normal lungs. However, when raised in the normal environment, the knockout mice had an increased incidence of lung infections. When these leaky *CFTR* knockouts were challenged with aerosolized bacteria, they were less able to clear the bacteria from their lungs than were normal controls, and repeated challenges led to classic CF lung disease. The conclusions from these studies are that the lung disease of CF results from repeated infections by organisms that are ineffectively cleared from the lung and that in the absence of infection, CF does not by itself result in lung disease. The implications of this study, if confirmed in humans, are profound. This means that the focus of research in CF will shift to examining the mechanisms by which the normal airway and the airway in CF patients deal with inhaled organisms, the differences in host defenses and, perhaps, the differences in the normal and CF inflammatory response. These are all new areas of research that hold great promise for the future. At the moment, it would appear that if CF patients were kept in a controlled environment, much the way the original gene therapy patients with severe combined immune deficiency disease were, they would not die of lung disease.

## Genetic Engineering of Human Proteins: Molecular Biology Versus Viscid Sputum

Cells make many thousands of proteins and, with rare exception, each protein accounts for only a small percentage of the cell's products. It is technically difficult and highly inefficient to attempt to collect large amounts of a specific protein for human use from normal cells. Enter molecular biology with its seemingly endless bag of tricks. Using recombinant DNA technology, one can induce cells to make large amounts of the protein of choice, and if this protein is secreted, it can be collected and purified for human use. This has been done for human insulin, growth hormone, tissue plasminogen activator, and factor VIII; recently, recombinant human DNase I has become available to treat patients with CF.

Respiratory disease in CF patients is characterized by accumulation of thick, purulent, tenacious sputum, filled with white blood cells and cellular debris. This sputum is difficult to clear from airways, and altered airway clearance produced by viscid sputum is felt to be partially responsible for the repeated infections that characterize CF. It has been known for many years that DNA can accumulate in high concentrations in the purulent sputum of CF patients and the degraded DNA no doubt contributes to the viscid nature of CF sputum. DNase I is a secreted enzyme that digests extracellular DNA. In the 1950s, bovine DNase I was approved for use by aerosol in CF patients to decrease sputum viscosity and make it easier for patients to raise secretions. Although effective, occasional adverse respiratory reactions to inhaled enzyme occurred, either because of allergic reactions to the foreign protein or to contaminating proteases that were present in the product, and this led to the halt in the use of DNase to thin the sputum of CF patients.

Again enter molecular biology, along with biotechnology, in the 1990s. The human DNase has now been cloned and expressed in a cell line, and the protein has been purified, its actions as a DNA-degrading enzyme confirmed, and its value as a clinical tool tested in a randomized, double-blind nationwide trial. Used as an aerosol either once or twice daily, the genetically engineered human DNase I (rhDNase) "reduced but did not eliminate exacerbations of respiratory symptoms, resulted in slight improvement in pulmonary function, and was well tolerated." Although the ultimate role of this form of therapy in CF remains to be determined and its cost-effectiveness needs to be proved (a single dose of rhDNase costs approximately $27), the emergence of this new form of therapy provides an opportunity to discuss the principles of genetically engineered proteins.

The first job in producing rhDNase was to find and clone the human gene (Fig. 6–8). To do this, a human pancreatic cDNA library was made by extracting RNA from the pancreas and by using the reverse transcriptase enzyme to convert mRNA to its complementary form, cDNA. The pancreas was chosen for the library because it produces the enzyme in abundance, and cDNA was chosen because the goal was to express the protein, not study its regulation as one might do with a genomic DNA library. The library was screened (see Chapter 3), with an oligonucleotide probe that was constructed from the known amino acid sequence of the protein DNAse I. Plaques that hybridized with the probe were identified, cloned, and sequenced, and the human gene with its 260 amino acid open reading frame, which included a

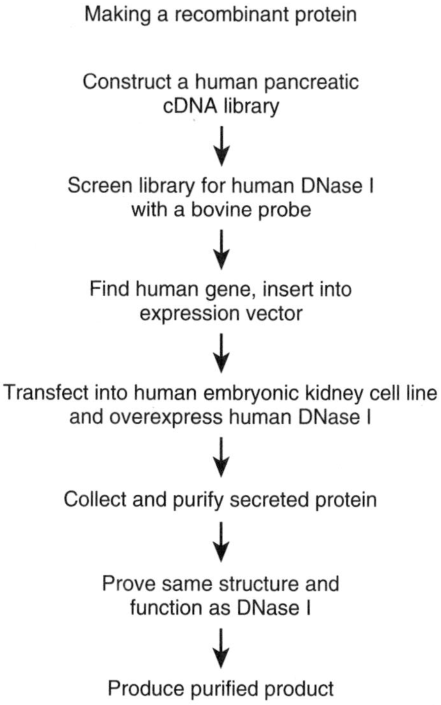

Making a recombinant protein

Construct a human pancreatic
cDNA library

↓

Screen library for human DNase I
with a bovine probe

↓

Find human gene, insert into
expression vector

↓

Transfect into human embryonic kidney cell line
and overexpress human DNase I

↓

Collect and purify secreted protein

↓

Prove same structure and
function as DNase I

↓

Produce purified product

FIGURE 6–8. **Making a recombinant protein.** The steps involved in making human DNAase I for human use. The first task was to find and clone the human gene by screening a pancreatic library for the cDNA. The gene was then inserted into a vector that provided for expression at a high level and allowed complete processing of the protein so that it was secreted. The protein could then be collected and purified and its structure and function verified and then tested as an agent that would liquefy secretions that had become thick and viscid as a result of free DNA.

signal peptide that allows synthesized proteins to be secreted, was in hand. The human cDNA was then placed in an expression vector, which is designed to produce large amounts of stable mRNA and to secrete the protein made from that mRNA. The vector for these studies had a strong viral promoter that served to drive overexpression of the human DNase enzyme (see Fig. 6–8). The vector was then transfected into a human kidney cell line, and transfected cells were selected by antibiotic resistance. The secreted protein was then isolated from the serum-free media and purified and its enzymatic activity tested.

One of the important issues in producing recombinant proteins is to pick the right cell line for transfection and protein production. Bacteria are cheap and easy to transfect but may not process the expressed protein in an appropriate fashion (e.g., glycosylate). Often this means that the protein does not fold appropriately to assume the structure that is necessary for its ultimate function. Viral vectors transfected into insect cells have overcome this problem to some extent, but it is generally felt that human cells are the best recipient for transfection of recombinant proteins to be used in humans.

Large amounts of human proteins are also being made for commercial purposes using the transgenic technology discussed in Chapter 3. However, these ventures employ two major variations of standard transgenic technology. First, larger animals are used: transgenic goats or cows. Second, the proteins being made must be secreted in some readily available form. Therefore, the transgene encoding the gene of interest is driven by a milk gene promoter such as the milk casein gene promoter. The transgenic protein is secreted in large amounts in milk; it is separated from the milk and purified and is ready for use. Of course the problem for CFTR is then how to get the protein to insert in the apical membrane of the airway epithelial cells so that it can function.

Many questions remain about CF and *CFTR*. Its exact function as a regulator of other ion channels must be worked out. The effect of various mutations on CFTR folding and resulting alterations in glycosylation of other proteins targeted for the cell surface, especially mucins, remains to be studied. Indeed correction of the folding defect may represent an important direction for future therapy. The role that *CFTR* plays in fetal lung development is not clear, even though it is expressed at higher levels than in the adult. The whole topic of gene therapy, of better targeting vectors, and of ways to deliver *CFTR* to submucosal glands, where its expression is highest, is being actively pursued.

## Gene Therapy for Cystic Fibrosis: The Promise and the Problems

The goal of gene therapy in CF is to target *CFTR* with sufficient efficiency to the appropriate cell types in the airway to functionally correct the ion transport defects that result in the respiratory diseases that lead to death. As discussed earlier, one might approach the problem by trying to get the CFTR protein to fold properly so that it can be transported to the cell surface, or one might attempt to bypass the CFTR and pharmacologically regulate other chloride or sodium channels. Indeed, one could manufacture the CFTR protein and attempt to have it taken up and transported to the apical cell surface of airway epithelial cells. However, the major focus of gene therapists has been to get the normal gene into the right cells in the most efficient fashion.

Although this sounds easy, it is not. Much has been done, much has been learned, but the task remains to be accomplished. The basic concepts of gene therapy and a detailed discussion of progress in this field appear in Chapter 5. Of course, much of the work on gene therapy has been done on CF cells and in CF patients. A quick summary of the state of the art as of the writing of this chapter is that the answer lies in finding a better vector. Virtually every vector has been used to transfect normal *CFTR*, and all of them work in cells and for a short time in fetal and adult animals. Two vectors have been tried in patients—adenoviral and liposomes. The report of the first clinical trial has just appeared, and the results were discouraging. Using an adenoviral vector instilled into the nose, investigators found evidence of gene transfer with low doses of virus but no change in the ion transport characteristics of the nasal mucosa. At high doses, nasal inflammation occurred. This type of inflammation has been found to be immune-mediated and to kill the very cells that express the transfected *CFTR*.

One direction that researchers have taken has been to attempt to modulate the immune response to the adenoviral vector. As noted before, adenoviral vectors, with the replicating elements removed, can efficiently target epithelial cells (airway cells express receptors for the virus) and can transfect nondividing cells. They do not integrate into the host genome so that they are not mutagenic. However, because they do not integrate, cells that turn over do not pass the gene on to daughter cells, and of course cells that die stop expressing the gene. Therefore, repeated transfections are needed. Repeated transfections generate the previously noted immune inflammatory response that abolishes transfected gene expression. This is a cellular and humoral immune response mediated by cytotoxic T cells; in particular TH2 helper T cells that activate IgA antiadenoviral antibodies. Recently, a group of investigators reasoned that if they stimulated TH1 helper cells at the expense of TH2 cells, the IgA-mediated immune response might be suppressed. They instilled into the trachea or gave intraperitoneally IL-12 or interferon-$\gamma$ at the time of gene transfection. The transient immune suppression of the TH2 T-cell subset worked, and the animals tolerated repeated transfections of adenovirus and expressed the transfected *CFTR* for longer periods than did controls. This type of transient and selective immune suppression does not carry the risk of more classic immune-modulating agents and holds some promise for the future.

## SUGGESTED READING

### General References

Crystal RG (ed): Cystic fibrosis—from the gene to the cure. Am J Respir Crit Care Med 151(Suppl):S45–S87, 1995.

### Identifying the Cystic Fibrosis Gene

Collins FS, Drumm ML, Cole JL, et al: Construction of a general human chromosome jumping library, with application to cystic fibrosis. Science 235:1046–1049, 1987.

Kerem B, Rommens JM, Buchanan JA, et al: Identification of the cystic fibrosis gene: Genetic analysis. Science 245:1073–1080, 1989.

Riordan JR, Rommens JM, Kerem B, et al: Identification of the cystic fibrosis gene: Cloning and characterization of complementary DNA. Science 245:1066–1072, 1989.

Roberts L: The race for the cystic fibrosis gene. Science 240:141–144; 282–285, 1988.

Rommens JM, Iannuzzi MC, Kerem B, et al: Identification of the cystic fibrosis gene: Chromosome walking and jumping. Science 245:1059–1065, 1989.

### *CFTR* Mutations

Highsmith WE, Burch LH, Zhou Z, et al: A novel mutation in the cystic fibrosis gene in patients with pulmonary disease but normal sweat chloride concentrations. N Engl J Med 331:974–980, 1994.

Welsh MJ, Smith AE: Molecular mechanisms of CFTR chloride channel dysfunction in cystic fibrosis. Cell 73:1251–1254, 1993.

Wine JJ: How do *CFTR* mutations cause cystic fibrosis? Curr Biol 5:1357–1359, 1995.

### DNase

Fuchs HJ, Borowitz DS, Christiansen DH, et al: Effect of aerosolized recombinant human DNase on exacerbations of respiratory symptoms and on pulmonary function in patients with cystic fibrosis. N Engl J Med 331:637–642, 1994. [accompanying editorial]

Shak S, Capon DJ, Hellmiss R, et al: Recombinant human DNase I reduces the viscosity of cystic fibrosis sputum. Proc Natl Acad Sci USA 87:9188–9192, 1990.

### The First *CFTR* Knockouts

Dorin JR, Dickinson P, Atton EW, et al: Cystic fibrosis in the mouse by targeted insertional mutagenesis. Nature 359:211–215, 1992.

Imundo L, Barasch J, Prince A, et al: Cystic fibrosis epithelial cells have a receptor for pathogenic bacteria on their apical surface. Proc Natl Acad Sci USA 92:3019–3023, 1995.

Snouwaert JN, Brigman KK, Latour AM, et al: An animal model for cystic fibrosis made by gene targeting. Science 257:1083–1088, 1992. [accompanying editorial]

Zhou L, Dey CR, Wert SE, et al: Correction of lethal intestinal defect in a mouse model of cystic fibrosis by human *CFTR*. Science 266:1705–1708, 1994.

### Gene Therapy

Knowles MR, Hohneker KW, Zhou Z, et al: A controlled study of adenoviral-vector-mediated gene transfer in the nasal epithelium of patients with cystic fibrosis. N Engl J Med 333:823–831, 1995. [accompanying editorial]

See also SUGGESTED READING in Chapter 5.

# Lung Cancer: DNA Synthesis and Repair, the Cell Cycle, and What Can Go Wrong

## The Nobel Prize, Molecules of the Year but Little Change in Survival (Yet)

Lung cancer is the number one cancer in men, continues to increase in incidence in women, and is the leading cause of cancer-related death in both sexes. Our knowledge about the cell cycle and its control and about the genetic mutations associated with cancer in general, and lung cancer in particular, has increased logarithmically over the past decade. The Nobel Prize was given for the discovery of oncogenes and their role in cancer. Two new classes of genes— growth suppression genes and the genes responsible for the repair of damaged DNA—have been implicated in cancer and have been designated "Molecules of the Year" in *Science* for 1994 and 1995, respectively. The new field of programmed cell death and its role in cancer has evolved. New approaches to the early diagnosis of lung cancer are being tested, and innovative approaches to the treatment of cancer, including gene therapy, are appearing at an ever-increasing rate. Indeed, the majority of human gene therapy trials now in progress involve the treatment of cancer patients, rather than the replacement of genes in patients with hereditary diseases. Although none of these scientific advances has yet had an impact on survival statistics, lung cancer provides an opportunity for this chapter to discuss a number of molecular biologic concepts and methods.

## DNA Synthesis: S Phase of the Cell Cycle

To understand the rapid and exciting advances that have occurred in the past 20 years in our knowledge of the pathophysiology, diagnosis, and treatment of disordered cell growth associated with lung cancer, one must first review the process of normal DNA replication and normal regulation of the cell cycle. The cell cycle is divided into four phases during which very different events occur (Figs. 7–1 and 7–2). M phase, or mitosis, represents the period of actual cell division in which duplicated chromosomes are segregated and the cell is pinched off into two daughter cells that contain exact duplicates of cellular DNA. M phase usually takes only 1 to 2 hours, whereas the rest of the cell cycle (also called interphase) takes 24 to 36 hours. Thus much of importance goes on in interphase. One crucial event is DNA synthesis, which results in complete replication of the genome. This occurs in S phase, which usually takes 6 to 10 hours. Each time that a cell divides, all the DNA within that cell is duplicated. Thus, prior to mitosis (actual cell division), two complete copies of all the DNA within that cell exist. DNA duplication

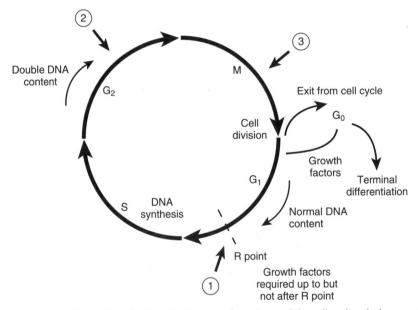

FIGURE 7–1. **The Cell Cycle: Part 1.** There are four phases of the cell cycle, which are not of equal length. The normal DNA content of cells in $G_0$ and $G_1$ increases in S phase when DNA is being replicated, is twice normal in $G_2$, and returns to normal in $G_0$ and $G_1$ after cells have divided. Growth factors are required to move the cell out of $G_0$ and to get the cell to the restriction point (R point). Thereafter, growth factors may be removed, and the cell will continue to move through the remainder of the cell cycle. The numbers in circles represent checkpoints that provide opportunities to determine (1) if all conditions for DNA synthesis have been met, (2) if DNA has been copied with fidelity, and (3) if the conditions for actual cell division are correct.

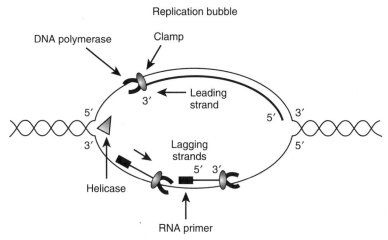

FIGURE 7–2. **DNA Synthesis and the Replication Fork-Bubble.** DNA synthesis begins at a number of places throughout the genome called replication origins. At these sites, proteins bind and open the DNA helix. Led by a helicase, which unwinds, and other proteins that hold apart the single strands of DNA, DNA polymerase (which is clamped to the DNA) slides along the original DNA strand in a 5′ to 3′ direction, adding nucleotides to the complementary leading strand, which is continuous. On the other strand, called the lagging strand because DNA synthesis must wait for the helicase moving ahead of the leading strand to provide single-stranded DNA for replication, DNA synthesis also moves in a 5′ to 3′ direction. Lagging strands begin with DNA primase synthesis of an RNA primer starting each short polymerase-catalyzed segment of new DNA. Lagging strands of DNA are synthesized until the polymerase runs into the RNA primer in front of it. The primers are then erased, and the ends of the short lagging strand segments of DNA are ligated together to form the new complementary DNA strand.

requires a series of complex processes that involve unwinding the DNA double helix and its interaction with DNA polymerase to produce two new strands of complementary DNA according to the base-pairing rules discussed in Chapter 1.

The first step in DNA replication requires breaking the H bonds between bases, leaving single-stranded DNA free to act as a template for new complementary DNA strands (see Fig. 7–2). DNA synthesis is initiated at special places in DNA called replication origins, where separation of the two strands is associated with formation of a replication bubble in which the DNA assembly machine functions. Several enzymes are involved in this process. They include helicase enzymes, which unwind the DNA helix and hold the two DNA strands apart, and DNA polymerases, which lock onto the DNA template and catalyze the addition of complementary bases to form new DNA chains. Ligases then patch pieces of the newly formed DNA together. DNA replication, which requires adenosine triphosphate as an energy source, proceeds at a rate of 40 to 50 nucleotides per second, but the fact that it proceeds simultaneously at many points along the 23 chromosomes allows the complete genome of $10^9$ base pairs to be duplicated during the 6 to 10 hours of S phase. The whole copying process usually occurs with very few errors, in part because any nucleotide not added at the 3′ end of the newly formed DNA chain is automatically clipped off.

## The Rest of the Cell Cycle and Its Regulation

The remaining portions of interphase are called $G_1$ and $G_2$; they precede and follow S phase, respectively. Each of these phases not only prepares for the next part of the cell cycle but also provides an opportunity to check the replication process; whether the cell is ready to undergo DNA replication (see 1 in Fig. 7–1), whether DNA has been faithfully copied (see 2 in Fig. 7–1), and whether conditions are optimal for cell division (see 3 in Fig. 7–1).

Cells also temporarily or permanently leave the cell cycle, moving into a quiescent phase called $G_0$. Some of these cells, and this is likely the case for alveolar type 2 cells and bronchiolar Clara cells, can be induced to move back into $G_1$ and thus re-enter the cell cycle, whereas other cells such as alveolar type 1 cells and airway ciliated cells permanently exit the cell cycle and lose the ability to replicate. Those cells that cannot re-enter the cell cycle or exit $G_0$ are said to be terminally differentiated. The processes that control terminal differentiation and entrance into and exit from $G_0$ are not well characterized.

There are a number of ways to determine at which point cells are in the cell cycle. DNA synthesis (S phase) can be monitored by assessing the uptake of radioactive thymidine or incorporation of a nonradioactive analog of thymidine, bromodeoxyuridine, into DNA, either biochemically or by visualization of cell or tissue sections. The amount of DNA in a cell can be assayed by staining cells with a dye that becomes fluorescent in a quantitative fashion when bound to DNA. One can then measure with a laser flow cytometer the number of cells having normal or twice-normal amounts of DNA. Cells in $G_0$ or $G_1$ have a single complement of DNA, whereas cells in $G_2$ or M have a double complement of DNA (see Fig. 7–1). Cells that are in S phase, making DNA, have an intermediate amount of DNA. In addition, the recent discovery of cyclin-dependent kinases (CDKs) (see later) and DNA-binding proteins such as the retinoblastoma protein (RB) that are activated during a precise point in the cell cycle, provide biochemical markers of the various stages of the cell cycle.

As noted earlier, there are a number of control points that operate in a feedback fashion to determine whether it is appropriate to proceed and trigger the events that lead to the next phase of the cell cycle. The feedback signals come from both the cell and its external environment. There are both positive and negative regulators of the process that interact to form a complex set of events whose accurate function ensures orderly cell proliferation and whose malfunction is the basis of cancer cell biology.

Most of what we know about mammalian cell cycle control was first explored in yeast, frog eggs, and other lower organisms. These organisms have simple and well-defined genetics (in the case of yeast) or can be easily grown, producing large amounts of protein (in the case of frog eggs). It is clear that much of the regulation of cell proliferation has been highly conserved throughout evolution. There are two major proteins that actively regulate the proteins actually involved in cell proliferation: (1) CDKs, which phosphorylate selected cell cycle proteins and (2) cyclins, which control the ability of CDKs to phosphorylate their targets by binding the CDKs (Fig. 7–3). Cyclins, which are synthesized and degraded in a cyclic process associated with the cell cycle, tend to fall into two classes: $G_1$ cyclins, which drive the cell into S phase and $G_2$ cyclins, which when activated drive the cell into M phase. Each set of cyclins binds specific CDKs, forming a complex that phosphorylates other key regulatory proteins.

One of the important targets of the cyclin-CDK complex is a group of pocket proteins, so called because their tertiary structure creates a pocket to

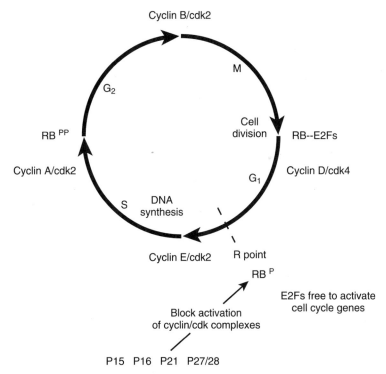

FIGURE 7–3. **The Cell Cycle: Part 2.** When activated, the complexes of cyclins and cyclin-dependent kinases (CDKs) phosphorylate pocket proteins such as RB, freeing the E2F family of transcriptional activators so that they can induce genes essential for progression through the cell cycle. Different cyclin/CDK complexes function at different parts of the cell cycle. A number of newly described proteins, P15, P21, and so on, block activation of different cyclin-CDK complexes, thereby acting as growth suppression genes. RB, by binding E2F, also acts as a growth suppression gene.

which cell cycle–related transcription factors, called E2Fs, bind (Fig. 7–4). The prototype of the pocket proteins is RB1 (the retinoblastoma protein), although there are at least two other pocket proteins, p107 and p130, whose names derive from their molecular weight. Unphosphorylated pocket proteins bind cell cycle–activating transcription factors. When they are phosphorylated by the cyclin-CDK complexes during different portions of the cell cycle, they release the transcription factors they have bound, and these factors then induce expression of important cell cycle genes, such as many of the enzymes involved in DNA synthesis. As the cell cycle proceeds, the pocket proteins again become dephosphorylated and rebind the transcription factors, turning off the genes they have activated. RB1 clearly is involved in the $G_1$ transition, whereas other pocket proteins may regulate different cell cycle transition

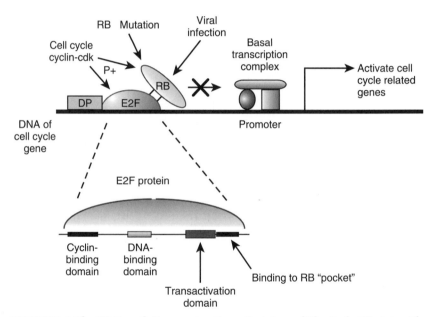

FIGURE 7–4. **The *RB* Growth Suppression Gene: Prototype of The Pocket Proteins.** The RB protein and other pocket proteins bind to E2F transcription factors, preventing them from transactivating important cell cycle–related genes. There is some evidence that the RB-E2F complex also acts as a repressor of gene expression. E2F is shown binding to the 5′ flanking region of a gene along with its partner DP. In this diagram, RB prevents E2F contact with the transcription complex of such a gene. RB and E2F are both phosphorylated by cyclin-CDK complexes. RB dissociates from E2F during the normal cell cycle (when phosphorylated by cyclin-CDKs), in viral infections (when viral proteins compete with E2Fs for RB), and when RB is mutated in cancer (when it is either deleted or is incapable of binding E2F). Under normal circumstances, RB binding to E2F, and therefore its growth suppression effect, is determined by the state of RB phosphorylation. The E2F proteins (there are now at least five of them) have a cyclin-binding domain, which provides a means of phosphorylating the E2F-DP complex; a DNA binding domain, which determines which genes they activate; a transactivating domain, which is the part of E2F that interacts with the basal transcription complex; and an RB-binding domain, which binds to the RB (or other family members) binding pocket.

points. Thus, the pocket proteins are called growth suppression genes because they suppress cell proliferation by binding to proteins that, when free, foster cell proliferation.

There is another, newly discovered, group of growth suppression genes that encode a series of proteins—p15, p16, p21, p27/p28 (the number of these proteins continues to grow)—that prevent activation of different cyclin-CDK complexes (see Fig. 7–3). Finally, there is another important growth suppression gene, *P53*, which interferes with cell cycle progression in a number of ways and appears to be an important checkpoint protein that recognizes DNA damage and determines whether DNA repair occurs or whether a cell undergoes apoptosis (Fig. 7–5).

## Balance of Positive and Negative Regulators of the Cell Cycle: Oncogenes and Growth Suppression Genes

There are many proteins that positively regulate cell proliferation, for example, growth factors, their receptors, and the signaling molecules that determine the appropriate nuclear response; the nuclear transcription factors regulating genes involved in moving the cell through the cell cycle; and the cyclins and their CDK partners. These positively acting proteins are balanced by the

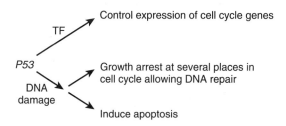

Many mutations in cancer

May act as an oncogene

May lose ability to induce apoptosis

May lose ability to arrest growth

FIGURE 7–5. **P53, the Multifunctional Growth Suppression Gene.** *P53* acts as a transcription factor that activates other genes (such as *P21*) that regulate the cell cycle. In addition, *P53* monitors DNA damage, inducing growth arrest at several places in the cell cycle. *P53* also appears to be essential for most forms of apoptosis. A large number of *P53* mutations have been described in cancer. With some mutations, *P53* actually functions as an oncogene. With others, *P53* loses its ability to induce growth arrest or apoptosis.

growth suppression genes noted in the preceding paragraph (Fig. 7–6). Errors that occur in the process of DNA synthesis are repaired by the newly discovered mismatch repair genes. Finally, cells that escape the repair process do not pass the stringent cell cycle checkpoints or receive conflicting growth signals and undergo a regulated process of cell suicide called apoptosis.

Tumor cells free themselves from the normal control of cell proliferation as a result of genetic changes that inappropriately activate the growth-promoting factors, inactivate the growth suppression factors, or interfere with the repair and cell death pathways. Any positively acting factor that functions inappropriately or in an uncontrolled fashion to drive the cell through the cell cycle is called an oncogene. These same factors acting in a normal fashion are called proto-oncogenes. The concept of proto-oncogenes and their oncogenic counterparts in transformed cells was first formulated by Bishop and Varmus in the 1970s. Some 70 positively acting oncogenes have been described in human tumors to date.

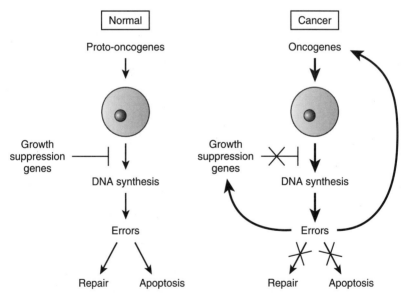

FIGURE 7–6. **Regulation of the Cell Cycle in Normal Cells and in Cancer: An Overview.** In normal cells, cell proliferation is regulated by signal-transducing proto-oncogenes and growth suppression genes. The fidelity of replicated DNA is monitored and errors are corrected by mismatch repair genes and by regulators of the apoptosis, or programmed cell death, pathway. In cancer, mutations or deletions, or both, have been described in each of these steps. Proto-oncogenes undergo mutations that result in their being overexpressed or constitutively expressed. Growth suppression genes are deleted or otherwise inactivated. Parts of the DNA repair system may become nonfunctional, and the apoptosis pathway may not be available. Errors in any one of these steps ultimately lead to an accumulation or errors at other steps, with invasive cancers often involving multiple gene defects.

## Oncogenes: Cancer in the 1970s and 1980s

Proto-oncogenes encompass any of the genes associated with signals that drive the cell through the cell cycle. They are, in the broad sense, signal-transducing proteins (Fig. 7–7). What types of mutations have been found in cancer and how do they activate growth-promoting oncogenes? Figure 7–8 depicts several types of gene mutations associated with cancer, and Figure 7–9 illustrates the point in the signal transduction cascade at which these mutations might lead to uncontrolled cell proliferation. This figure also lists some of the oncogenes that have been associated with lung cancer.

Point mutations (discussed in depth in Chapter 3) have been described as the cause for constitutive (unregulated) activation of *ras* in many tumors (see Fig. 7–8). Structural homology to G proteins is possessed by ras proteins; thus they play a role in transducing growth factor signals. Mutations in *ras* have been described in non–small-cell lung cancers (NSCLCs), especially adenocarcinomas, but not in small-cell lung cancers (SCLCs). Activated *ras,* or activation of other signal-transducing proteins, drives cell proliferation in a growth factor–independent fashion.

Chromosomal translocations join pieces of a chromosome containing a proto-oncogene to a piece of another chromosome that regulates a different gene. When the gene is a constitutively active gene (is always being tran-

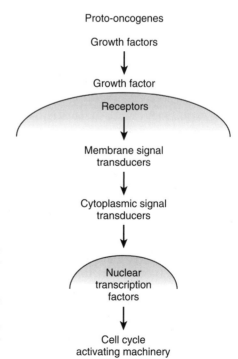

FIGURE 7–7. **Proto-oncogenes: Signal Transduction from Cell Surface to DNA.** Proto-oncogenes are any part of the signaling system that regulates cell proliferation, from the growth factor ligands that bind to specific cell surface receptors to the downstream signaling molecules that activate the nuclear cell cycle machinery that results in cell proliferation.

Proto-oncogene to oncogene

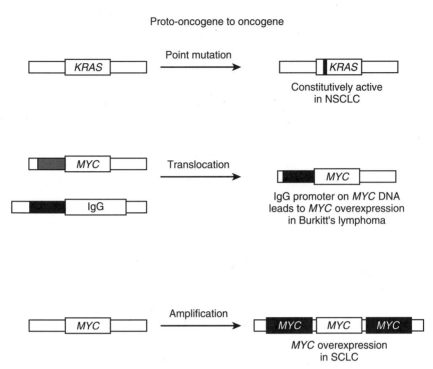

FIGURE 7–8. **Proto-oncogene to Oncogene Mutations.** See text for explanation. The black areas represent mutations that result in activation of oncogenes in cancer. In each instance, the mutation results in overexpression of the proto-oncogene, which then becomes an oncogene.

scribed) such as the IgG gene, the proto-oncogene is overexpressed and becomes an oncogene, driving the cell in which it is expressed through the cell cycle. Such translocation has been described for *myc* in Burkitt's lymphoma, and for Bcl-2, a protein that rescues cells from apoptosis. Overexpression of Bcl-2 would allow cells that have accumulated mutations to live when they otherwise would have entered the programmed cell death pathway.

Genes may be present in many copies—a mutation called gene amplification. Amplification of *myc* has been described in many tumors, and *myc* family transcription factors, L-myc and N-myc, have been found to be amplified in SCLC. Activated genes require that only one allele be affected, that is, they are dominant genes. The resultant overproduction of the mutant proto-oncogene, now an oncogene, is sufficient to alter the cell cycle. However, it has been shown that a single oncogene cannot by itself cause cell transformation. Such transformation is defined by the ability of cells to form tumors when injected into mice, in addition to the loss of many cell growth controls. It requires mutations and therefore overexpression of at least two oncogenes. Although more than 70 oncogenes have been described in human tumors, such dominant mutations have been found in only 20% of cancers.

Oncogenes in lung cancer

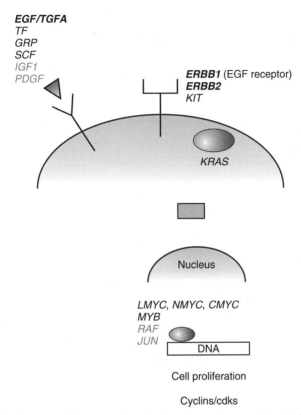

FIGURE 7–9. **Oncogene Mutations Described in Lung Cancers.** Growth factors, growth factor receptors, signal transduction, nuclear transcription factors, and cell proliferation gene mutations that have been described in lung cancer are presented. Those in bold have been found exclusively or predominantly in non–small-cell lung cancer (NSCLC), those in black in small-cell lung cancer (SCLC), and those in light italics in both.

## Growth Suppression Genes: Cancer in the 1980s and 1990s

If the 1970s was the era of oncogenes, the 1980s and 1990s have been the era of growth suppression genes. The possibility that growth suppression genes play a role in cancer was first noted in cell fusion experiments in which transformed cells were fused with normal cells. After fusion, the transformed cells displayed normal growth regulation for a number of cell cycles, as if something that had been deleted from these cells was supplied by fusion with the normal cells. Later it was noted that viruses associated with cancer—for example, the papillomavirus in cervical cancer—bind to and inactivate the two major growth suppression proteins, RB and P53. Several adenoviral genes are also capable of binding to RB and P53 and displacing E2F transcription factors, thereby removing the normal inhibition against cell proliferation. This is the mechanism used by viruses to propagate in cells. Finally, it has been shown that transfection of cells with portions of the genes that bind to RB and P53, abolishes their growth suppression activity and immortalizes normal cells.

Mutations in growth suppression genes are now being found in many human tumors. These are recessive rather than dominant mutations, requiring that both alleles be altered before the gene is inactivated because absence of a protein, rather than an excess of protein, produces dysregulation of the cell cycle. Most forms of hereditary cancer involve deletions or mutations of growth suppression genes, or both. The classic example of hereditary cancer, and the paradigm for the growth suppression gene concept, first elucidated by Knudson, which has now been extended to many other cell cycle regulators, involves the retinoblastoma gene (see earlier discussion of cell cycle regulation and also Fig. 7–10). In individuals with a family history of retinoblastoma, there is an inherited (germ line) deletion of *RB*. If the deletion is inherited from both parents, death of the embryo occurs (an embryonic lethal mutation). However, if only one allele is missing, a subsequent second mutation in a somatic cell leads to uncontrolled cell growth in that specific tissue. Such somatic mutations occur with high frequency in the retina, which is subject to DNA damage from light, and since only retinal cells have lost or inactivated both *RB* alleles, tumors (retinoblastomas) develop only in the retina. In fact, individuals with hereditary retinoblastoma do have a high incidence of tumors (implying second mutations) elsewhere in the body, especially osteosarcomas. However, tumors with *RB* deletions also occur in individuals with no family history. In this case, it is presumed that two somatic mutations are required, since the individual is born with two normal RB alleles. *RB* mutations have been found with high frequency in lung cancer. As many as 60% of individuals with SCLCs and 10% of individuals with NSCLCs have been found to have *RB* deletions and 75% of the remaining SCLC patients have abnormal RB protein that does not phosphorylate or bind E2F transcription factors.

A similar picture has been developed for the P53 protein, which is absent or inactive in 75% of SCLC patients and in 50% of NSCLC patients. The *P53* hereditary syndrome that is comparable to the RB story is the Li-Fraumeni syndrome (Table 7–1). Other recessive growth suppression genes are the *APC* gene (adenoma polyposis coli) found in patients with hereditary polyposis and in a large number of patients with colon cancer. Another such recessive gene is discussed in detail later in this chapter. It is a DNA mismatch repair enzyme that is found to be defective in 50 to 60% of individuals with a hereditary form of colon cancer not associated with polyps and in 15% of nonhereditary forms of colon cancer. Recent studies of lung cancer patients have suggested that one of the proteins (P16) that blocks activation of a cyclin-CDK complex that phosphorylates RB may be absent in the majority

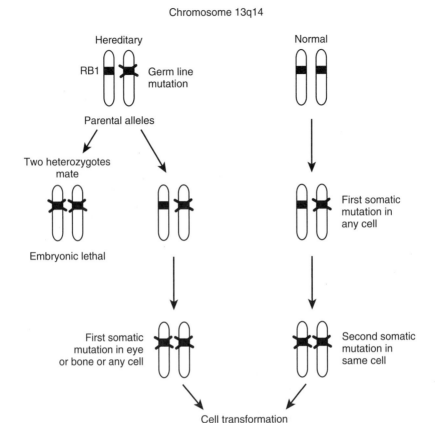

FIGURE 7–10. **Retinoblastoma Gene Deletions: A Model for All Growth Suppression Gene Mutations.** The *RB* gene is located on chromosome 13q. In hereditary retinoblastoma, one parent carries a deleted RB allele. If this allele is passed on via germ cells to an offspring, that person will have only one functional *RB* gene in all cells. If that lone *RB* gene is mutated in the eye, retinoblastoma will develop; if it is mutated in bone, osteosarcoma will form. If both parents are heterozygous for retinoblastoma and pass the deleted allele to the offspring, the embryo will die in utero. In nonhereditary settings, all cells carry *RB* on both chromosomes. If first one allele is mutated and then a second mutation occurs in the same cell, transformation will occur.

of NSCLCs. This gene is also deleted in familial melanomas and in pancreatic adenocarcinomas. Table 7–1 lists a number of growth suppression genes whose deletions have been associated with cancer.

How do all these recessive mutations occur? Breaks in chromosomes that are not repaired lead to large deletions that can be recognized on

TABLE 7–1
*Putative Growth Suppression Genes Implicated In Cancer*

| Gene | Chromosome | Disease | Function |
|------|-----------|---------|----------|
| MSH2 | 2p16 | HNPCC (colon cancer) | Mismatch repair |
| PMS1 | 2q31 | | Mismatch repair |
| MLH1 | 3p21 | | Mismatch repair |
| VHL | 3p26 | von Hippel-Lindau disease | Rate of transcription |
| APC | 5q21 | Adenoma polyposis coli | Cell adhesion |
| PMS2 | 7p22 | | Mismatch repair |
| P21 | 6p21 | | Suppress cyclin-CDK |
| P16 | 9p21 | Familial melanoma | Suppress cyclin-CDK |
| P15 | 9p21 | | Suppress cyclin-CDK |
| WT-1 | 11p13 | Wilms' tumor | |
| RB | 13p14 | Retinoblastoma | Suppress transcription |
| P53 | 17p13 | Li-Fraumeni syndrome | Multiple |
| BRCA2 | 13q | Breast cancer | |
| BRCA1 | 17q21 | Breast cancer | |
| NF1 | 17q11 | Neurofibroma | |
| DCC | 18 | Colon cancer | Cell adhesion |
| NF2 | 22q | Meningioma | |

HNPCC, hereditary nonpolyposis colon cancer gene.

cytogenetic preparations of chromosomes. However, most deletions associated with cancer are microdeletions of small areas of chromosomal DNA that cannot be recognized by visual examination of chromosomes. Although the mechanisms responsible for gene deletions in cancer have not been completely defined, mitotic recombination can occur. This is similar to the meiotic recombination responsible for crossover exchange of genetic information between chromosomes (see Fig. 4–1). Mitotic recombination rarely occurs normally, but DNA damage induced by radiation (and likely other DNA-damaging agents) increases the frequency of mitotic recombination and the possibility of losing pieces of DNA. Of course, all the DNA mutations associated with loss of proteins that are illustrated in Chapter 3 can occur. Point, missense, and nonsense mutations, along with altered splice sites, can eliminate or alter the function of the normal protein.

Recently, another form of gene inactivation associated with impaired transcription of DNA into RNA has been described for the P16 protein in cell lines and in primary tumors of patients with NSCLC. As noted earlier, P16 is one of the proteins that blocks activation of a cyclin-CDK complex. Its absence has been implicated in a variety of cancers, but sequencing of the *P16* gene in these cancers has often failed to define specific mutations. This lack of DNA mutations in the *P16* gene led a group of investigators to ask whether, even though *P16* DNA was normal, the problem might not be with transcription of the DNA with consequent absence of the P16 mRNA and protein. Chapters 1 and 8 discuss regulation of gene transcription. One possibility for the inability to transcribe normal DNA is that normal transcription factors may not be available or may be mutated so that they do not activate *P16* transcription. Another possibility for impaired transcription is that *P16* DNA binding sites for transcription factors are not available. Methylation of CpG islands in genomic DNA is involved in the regulation of cell differentiation during development and has recently been implicated in cancer. A large percentage of the cytosines in CG nucleotide sequences of vertebrate DNA are methylated. The presence of the methyl group tends to make the DNA inaccessible to the binding of transcription factors. The patterns of CpG methylation tend to be inherited, and they determine which genes are active or inactive in a particular cell. CpG methylation is determined after the early stages of development by an enzyme called maintainance methylase. It has long been thought that *hypomethylation* may be a mechanism by which oncogenes are turned on; that is, lack of normal CpG methylation allows binding of transcription factors and constitutive expression of proto-oncogenes that are normally transcriptionally inactive. Recent studies suggest that *hypermethylation* of growth suppression genes may be an important mechanism for preventing transcription of important negative regulators of cell proliferation. This has proved to be the case in an animal model of HPCC (hereditary polyposis colon carcinoma, a hereditary form of colonic polyps) in which blocking methylation prevents the appearance of colon cancer. Now such a mechanism has been implicated in the absence of *P16* mRNA and protein in lung cancer. *P16* has a large CpG island in the regulatory region of its first exon (Fig. 7–11). This island is normally not methylated and therefore allows binding of transcription factors required to activate transcription of *P16*. However, in NSCLC cell lines and tumors, hypermethylation of this island occurs and the *P16* gene is not transcribed. As a result, there is no *P16* mRNA and no protein. In this instance, DNA mutations are not the reason that *P16* is absent, rather altered transcription of *P16* is the problem. The regulation of methylation and of methylase genes is now an active area of investigation in cancer biology.

## Progression of Genetic Mutations in Cancer: The Multiple Hit Hypothesis

It has become clear that there are many mutations, resulting in both gain and loss of function, in human tumors. Recent studies have suggested that cancer arises not from a single mutation but rather from an accumulation of mutations, which may be sequential in nature. This "multiple hit" hypothesis of cancer has been best characterized in colon cancer. It states that a single

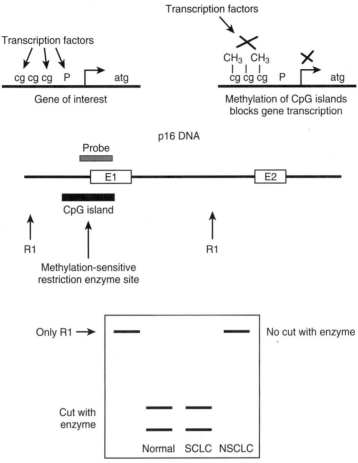

FIGURE 7–11. **Hypermethylation of CpG Islands Prevents Transcription of the Growth Suppression Gene *P16*.** Under normal circumstances, transcription factors bind to DNA in the 5′ flanking region of *P16* DNA and activate transcription of the gene (cg represent CpG islands, P = promoter). If hypermethylation of CpG islands occurs, the transcription factors do not bind and activate transcription, and the mRNA and protein are not produced. The restriction enzyme R1 cuts the *P16* DNA into one large piece. The methylation-sensitive enzyme cuts the normal *P16* DNA of SCLC into two smaller pieces, but fails to cut the hypermethylated DNA of a NSCLC.

mutation provides a cell a growth advantage. Second and third mutations provide additional growth advantages, which result in clonal (deriving from a single cell) tumor formation. Furthermore, each mutation not only provides a growth advantage but also increases the cell's susceptibility to subsequent mutations. Eventually, such cells accumulate sufficient dominant oncogene and recessive growth suppression gene mutations to become transformed and malignant, enabling them to invade tissues and metastasize. The multiple hit, accumulation of mutation hypothesis accounts for the increased incidence of tumors in older individuals and the long lag time between mutational insults such as radiation exposure and the actual appearance of tumors.

As noted earlier, the multiple hit hypothesis has been best studied in colon cancer. Investigators have correlated gene mutations over time in tissue biopsies as colonic polyps progress to highly malignant carcinomas (Fig. 7–12). The work was first performed in individuals with familial polyposis in which a deleted or inactivated gene (the *APC* gene) was identified in linkage analysis studies on the long arm of chromosome 5. Family members had a deleted or mutated APC allele in all cells (because it was inherited and existed in germ cells), analogous to the situation in hereditary retinoblastoma. It was subsequently found that 65 to 70% of individuals with nonhereditary polyps leading to colon cancer also had lost the *APC* gene. Studies of sequential biopsies of both types of patients defined a series of loss or gain of function mutations that appeared during the course of cell transformation (see Fig. 7–10).

Although many genetic abnormalities of both oncogenes and growth suppression genes have been described in lung cancer, there is no simple way of extending the multiple hit hypothesis to lung cancer, although the finding that some abnormalities (e.g., *myc*) are associated with poor prognosis suggests accumulation of mutations in lung cancer. No airway analog of familial polyposis exists, and biopsy specimens of resected lung cancers are surrounded by normal lung tissue, so it is difficult to detect allelic loss when a mix of tumor and normal lung tissue is analyzed. Histologic equivalents of progressive stages of cell transformation in the colon do exist in the lung; it is generally felt that epithelial cell hyperplasia proceeds to metaplasia, carcinoma in situ, and to frank squamous cell carcinoma. Similar histologic stages have not been as carefully defined for peripheral lung cancers. However,

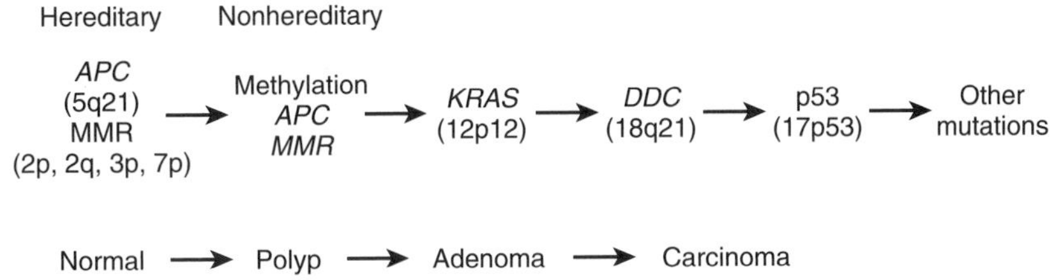

Hereditary    Nonhereditary

APC
(5q21)    →    Methylation
APC    →    KRAS
(12p12)    →    DDC
(18q21)    →    p53
(17p53)    →    Other
mutations
MMR
(2p, 2q, 3p, 7p)        MMR

Normal → Polyp → Adenoma → Carcinoma

FIGURE 7–12. **The Multi-Hit Sequence of Mutations in Colon Cancer.** The progress of normal colon to polyp to adenoma and ultimately to invasive cancer is charted; gene mutations that are associated with each stage of disease are listed at the top of the figure. In families with hereditary multiple polyposis coli or nonpolyposis colon cancer, the *APC* gene or mismatch repair (MMR) genes, respectively, are deleted in normal tissue. In nonhereditary disease, these abnormalities occur at the polyp stage. Thus growth suppression genes are affected first in colon cancer. The oncogene *K-ras* is activated and the growth suppression gene *DCC* is deleted at the adenoma stage. *P53* mutations, along with a variety of other mutations, occur late in invasive types of colon cancer. The numbers in parentheses are chromosomal locations of genes.

recent studies of human tissue obtained from surgical resections have begun to approach this problem. These studies have used microdissection of paraffin-embedded tissue to tease out several hundred pure populations of normal, hyperplastic, or carcinomatous cells for subsequent genetic analysis by polymerase chain reaction (PCR) techniques.

One recent study focused on deletions or loss of heterozygosity in several regions of chromosome 3p that are thought to contain growth suppression genes. When genetic deletions occur, areas that flank the gene of interest are also lost or replaced, with the consequence that the normal maternal-paternal heterozygosity for flanking DNA sequences is lost. Although each parental allele may carry the *RB* gene, the DNA in the immediate vicinity of the *RB* allele will not be identical because of human genetic diversity associated with meiotic recombination (see Fig. 4–1). Thus individuals are normally heterozygous (also called polymorphic) for much of their chromosomal DNA. When microdeletions occur for any of the previously noted reasons, not only will the gene of interest be lost but DNA surrounding this area can also be altered or lost. If one has probes for the area around the gene of interest or can perform PCR in this area with primers to known sequences, one can detect chromosomal loss of heterozygosity (Fig. 7–13). The human genome project (see Chapter 10) has produced detailed maps of each chromosome using primers that flank repeat sequences throughout the genome (see also discussion of microsatellites later). This approach has been used to detect areas on chromosomes that might contain tumor suppressor genes. Indeed, new tumor suppressor genes have been cloned guided by loss of heterozygosity using the positional cloning strategies discussed in Chapter 6.

By using these methods to analyze NSCLCs, investigators found that cells that were clearly invasive cancer cells had evidence of chromosome 3p allelic loss in most tumors (see Fig. 7–13). However, loss of heterozygosity was also noted when hyperplastic cells, which are presumably preneoplastic, away from the area of carcinoma were analyzed. Since normal lymphocytes in the area of cancer or completely normal lung cells demonstrated no loss of heterozygosity, these findings suggest that chromosome 3p allelic losses are early lesions similar to the *APC* gene defect in colon cancer. Allelic loss was observed in alveoli, bronchioles, and bronchi from tumor specimens, suggesting that lung cancer may be associated with a field defect, that is, mutagenesis of an entire area of lung rather than clonal growth of a single mutagenized cell.

This same group of investigators, using similar microdissection techniques, has shown that *K-ras* mutations that lead to activation of this oncogene are a late event in NSCLC, in contrast to the early appearance of chromosome 3p deletions. Although the mechanism of these chromosome 3p deletions is not clear (nor is it clear which specific genes might actually be affected), these studies have begun to establish a multiple hit sequence for NSCLC similar to that proposed for colon cancer.

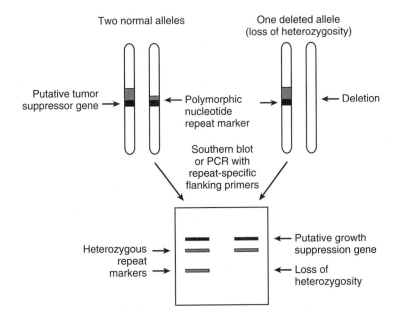

Sequential mutations in NSCLC

|  | Loss of heterozygosity (3p) (field defect) | KRAS mutations (clonal) |
|---|---|---|
| Normal | 0% | 0% |
| Hyperplasia | 76% | 0% |
| Dysplasia | 86% | 8% |
| Noninvasive | 100% | 8% |
| Invasive | 100% | 100% |

FIGURE 7–13. **Loss of Heterozygosity: Sequential Mutations in Lung Cancer.** The illustration depicts maternal and paternal chromosomes. Each has a putative tumor suppressor gene (black area). The di- or trinucleotide repeat marker *(gray shading)* is polymorphic, that is, it is a different length at each allele. When one allele is deleted, there is a loss of normal heterozygosity; now only one repeat is present. When this loss of heterozygosity is present in tumor tissue, it implies that the putative tumor suppressor gene is also deleted. Thus the loss of heterozygosity in tumor tissue focuses on an area of a possible tumor suppressor, although it does not actually identify the suppressor gene involved. When cells from NSCLC were analyzed, there was loss of heterozygosity at several places on chromosome 3p in hyperplastic, dysplastic, and actual tumor tissue. The loss of heterozygosity was observed in alveolar, bronchiolar, and bronchial cells, suggesting that mutations had occurred in a whole field or area, rather than in a single cell. In contrast, *K-ras* mutations were seen only in the latter stages of cell transformation. These data suggest that loss of tumor suppressor genes on chromosome 3p occurred early in lung cancer, whereas *K-ras* oncogene mutations occurred late. The exact locus of the chromosome 3p genes involved has not been determined (although there are several possible candidates on chromosome 3p), nor is it clear that the second (present) allele is also mutated. The latter must occur if the gene is to lose function.

## Cancer in the 1990s and into the Next Millennium: DNA Repair Defects

It is estimated that human cells go through a total of $2^{10}$ divisions in a lifetime. With each cell containing $3 \times 10^9$ base pairs and with the estimated error rate for DNA replication at about $10^{-10}$ mutations per base pair per cell generation, it is obvious that there is plenty of chance for mutations to occur within one's lifetime, even without exposure to environmental mutagens such as cigarette smoke or ultraviolet radiation. One of the reasons that DNA mutations do not rapidly accumulate is the DNA polymerase self-correcting system of making certain that bases are added only in the 5′ to 3′ fashion during DNA replication. However, as the preceding paragraphs attest, mutations do occur during cell proliferation. Correction of these mutations involves a number of recently described DNA repair enzymes whose importance, especially in the field of cancer biology, has earned the "Molecule of the Year" award for 1994 by *Science* magazine.

The DNA repair enzymes were first explored in bacteria, and it has only been in the past several years that their human counterparts have been identified and their potential role in cancer has been defined. The mismatch repair (MMR) genes recognize mismatches in replicating strands of DNA, excise the mismatched area, induce correct replication, and ligate in place the new correct segment of DNA (Fig. 7–14).

DNA can also be injured by environmental mutagens such as chemicals or radiation. Two pathways have been defined that are involved in repair of DNA errors and DNA damage. The base excision repair pathway targets single damaged bases. The nucleotide excision repair pathway recognizes large areas of mismatched or damaged DNA, unwinds the DNA, excises these areas, and replaces them with new DNA. Xeroderma pigmentosum, which is characterized by multiple skin cancers, is associated with defects in the nucleotide excision repair system.

However, it is the MMR system involving the so-called mutator genes that has attracted most cancer researchers. This system repairs mismatches that have eluded the base pairing rule of A-T and G-C. These mismatches most often occur within the long di-, tri-, and tetranucleotide repeats that appear frequently in genomic DNA and were discussed in Chapter 3. In this case, slippage of the copy strand of DNA often occurs, and one or several bases are not copied in sequence. Four genes involved in MMR and their encoded proteins have been discovered in humans to date (see Fig. 7–14). The failure of MMR function in these so-called microsatellite repeats provides a means of linkage analysis, as discussed in Chapter 3, since the length of microsatellites is polymorphic and inherited, differing on maternal and paternal alleles. However, failure of MMR function also provides a means of recognizing genetic instability, since defects in MMR genes mark cells via altered length of microsatellites (either shorter or longer) that have undergone mutations.

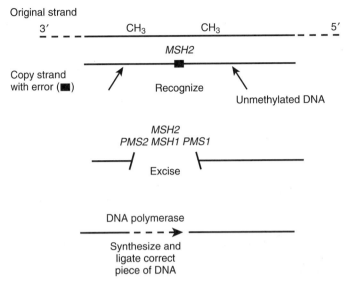

FIGURE 7–14. **Mismatch Repair: Recognizing the Wrong Sequence and Replacing It.** The original strand of DNA is methylated in various places, whereas the newly copied strand has not yet been methylated. The new strand has an extra nucleotide (black box) that has been incorrectly inserted. First, the MSH2 protein recognizes the mismatch on the nonmethylated strand. MSH1 then binds to MSH2 and together with the other proteins excises the segment containing the error. DNA polymerase then copies the correct DNA (dashed line) replacing the excised segment, and this new DNA is ligated in place.

The MMR defect in human cancer was first identified in a form of hereditary colon cancer not associated with polyposis (initially called the human nonpolyposis colon cancer gene—*HNPCC*). A deletion in chromosome 2 was noted in these individuals, and the deleted gene that was identified was homologous to one of the MMR genes that binds to the mismatched area of nucleotides in *Escherichia coli*. This deletion, of the human *MSH2* gene, was found in 50 to 60% of *HNPCC* individuals. A deletion of a second MMR gene, located on chromosome 3, the human *MSH1* gene, which binds to *MSH2* and excises the mismatched segment, accounted for an additional 30% of *HNPCC* cases. It is now known that 10 to 15% of sporadic colon cancers are associated with allelic loss of one of the four known human MMR genes. The MMR defects are recessive mutations, so a single normal allele is sufficient to provide normal MMR function. Therefore, both copies of MMR genes must be lost or mutated to predispose cells to genetic instability. In hereditary nonpolyposis colon carcinoma, one allele is missing in all cells, making all cells susceptible to a second mutation and defective repair. In nonhereditary disease, instability is found in cells in and around the tumor, but not in normal cells. Like retinoblastoma or patients with Li-Fraumeni syndrome, individuals with hereditary nonpolyposis colon carcinoma are at high risk for the development of cancers at many sites. The hypothesis is that defects in repairing DNA result in mutations in other cell cycle–related genes, ultimately leading to cell transformation.

Similar studies have begun to be carried out in lung cancer. The work noted earlier showing that deletions in chromosome 3p were present in early stages of NSCLC used microsatellite lengths as a way of finding allelic deletions and therefore diagnosing genetic instability. As noted earlier, *MSH1* is located on chromosome 3p (Fig. 7–15). A second study of microsatellite genetic instabiliy in lung cancer has applied PCR techniques using oligonucle-otide primers that flank known tri- and tetranucleotide repeats on seven different chromosomes. In this study, DNA was isolated from normal or tumor tissue by microdissection, as described previously, or from sputum or urine samples (in the case of bladder cancer). It was found that 9% of NSCLC and 50% of SCLC tissue exhibited microsatellite alterations for two or more markers. In those individuals in whom sputum samples were available, the same microsatellite alterations were noted in tumor and in sputum. Since the PCR primers were not chosen to reflect allelic deletions of a specific gene, and no chromosome dominated in the microsatellite alterations, these studies suggest generalized DNA instability such as might occur with MMR gene defects. This study also found defects at the margin of resection in several tumor samples, raising the question of whether this technique could be used to determine the appropriate site for tumor resections. Alternatively, and more likely in light of the previously discussed findings of chromosome 3p allelic deletions, the results could be used to support the field theory of generalized areas of DNA mutation. It seems likely that these methods will be increasingly applied to specific chromosomal areas subject to frequent mutations as both a diagnostic and prognostic tool.

## New Ways to Treat Cancer: The Real Venue of Gene Therapy

The previous discussion makes clear the fact that we have learned a great deal about the biology of cell proliferation and the molecular mechanisms involved in the control of this process. These multiple insights into the cell replication process have had little impact yet on the prevention of cancer or on longevity once cancer has been diagnosed. However, many new ideas for treatment are being tested in animals and humans with encouraging results. Several of these ideas are discussed in the following sections, partly because they have had clinical trials with some success and partly because they further illustrate general principles of molecular biology.

### SUICIDE GENES

One approach to killing tumor cells has involved the thymidine kinase selection system discussed in the section on gene knockout experiments in Chapter 4.

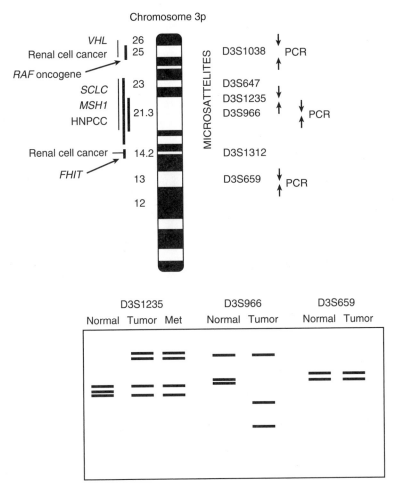

FIGURE 7–15. **Microsatellite Instability and Chromosome 3p.** Diagram of chromosome 3p, with relevant gene locations on the left and nucleotide repeat sequences on the right. Maps of the whole human genome covered by these repeats are now available so that any chromosome can be analyzed in this fashion. The repeats listed cover different areas of the chromosome, in areas around genes that may be causally involved in carcinogenesis. At the bottom of the figure are the results of polymerase chain reaction (PCR) amplification of tumor DNA using three different sets of primers that amplify three different repeat units. Using D3S1235, one can see that there are three repeats in normal tissue taken from areas away from the tumor or from normal lymphocytes, but that microsatellite instability in tumor and in a metastatic focus results in additional repeats of larger size. Using marker D3S966, instability is evident by the presence of multiple bands of smaller than normal size in the tumor. Marker D3S659 is the same; it demonstrates similar lengths of repeat elements in normal and tumor tissue. Whether results such as these indicate generalized genomic instability (which would also be accompanied by evidence of instability on other chromosomes) or indicates local chromosomal instability and possible mutations in the *VHL* or *MSH1* gene is not yet clear. Generalized instability might be expected in mismatch repair genes that have been mutated or deleted, whereas local instability might be expected if a single growth suppression gene were deleted.

Tumor cells are transfected with the herpes simplex thymidine kinase *(TK)* gene and animals bearing the tumor are given the nucleoside analog ganciclovir. Normally, ganciclovir is not toxic to mammalian cells but will kill cells that express the viral *TK* gene. *TK* transforms ganciclovir into a purine that can compete with normal nucleotides for incorporation into DNA in proliferating cells. This DNA is unstable, is degraded, and *TK*-expressing cells die. Thus, viral *TK* has been called a suicide gene. Other enzymes that aid in the activation of toxic drugs have also been used to aid in the killing of proliferating cells, but *TK* is the best studied of the suicide genes (Fig. 7–16).

The herpes *TK* gene has been injected into a variety of tumors using retroviral and more recently adenoviral vectors. In a number of individuals in whom brain tumors have been injected with this gene, significant tumor regression has occurred when ganciclovir is given. This approach requires that the tumor be localized and accessible, as in the case of brain tumors. Intuitively, it seems that all the tumor cells need to be transfected if the method is to be successful; however, this has not proved to be the case. There appears to be a "bystander effect" in which cells die even though they are not expressing the *TK* gene. Whether this results from release and then reuptake of *TK* by nontransfected cells or release of toxic substances by dying cells is not clear. Recent studies have extended the work in large focal tumors to more diffuse tumors in enclosed spaces. In this case, the *TK* gene has been transfected into peritoneal and pleural mesotheliomas or diffuse peritoneal

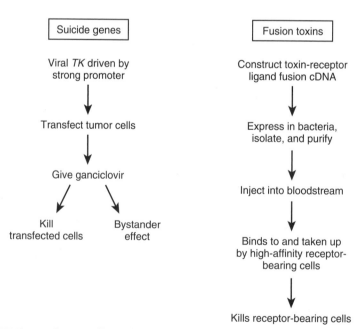

FIGURE 7–16. **Selective Killing of Cancer Cells: Suicide Genes and Fusion Toxins.** See text for explanation.

adenocarcinomas by washing these closed spaces with the *TK*-bearing vector. Although human studies are now in progress, this approach holds some hope (at least for palliation) in the treatment of these uniformly fatal types of cancer.

## MAGIC BULLETS: THE FUSION TOXINS

Usual forms of chemotherapy often kill normal as well as abnormal cells and as a result have many unwanted side effects. In addition, drug resistance ultimately limits the effectiveness of many of these agents. As a result, the search for better, more selective ways to kill cells continues. Selective cell killing can be accomplished by targeting cells that express a specific antigen with monoclonal antibodies or immune toxins. One novel approach has been to create fusion toxins (see Fig. 7–16), that is, engineer molecules that combine two or more proteins, one of which is toxic to cells and one of which targets specific cells. The toxins can be combined with molecules of the immune system that bind to specific receptors or with growth factors that bind to cells that uniquely express growth factor receptors. Diphtheria toxin is an effective killer of cells; a single molecule is capable of killing a cell. Recently, investigators produced a fusion toxin that combines the transmembrane and catalytic domains of diphtheria toxin with the receptor-binding domain of interleukin 2 (IL-2). This molecule, when injected intravenously, selectively binds to cells that express the high-affinity IL-2 receptor, and the molecule is then internalized via receptor-mediated endocytosis. The endocytic vesicle is acidified, releasing the toxin into the cytoplasm where the catalytic domain of the toxin inhibits protein synthesis, thereby killing the cell. Activated T and B lymphocytes and monocytes express the high-affinity IL-2 receptor and are thus targets for the fusion toxin. This approach is now being investigated as a therapy for cutaneous T-cell lymphoma, psoriasis, type 1 diabetes, and HIV-related diseases. One can obviously engineer a fusion toxin with growth factors that would target cells expressing high levels of epidermal growth factor (EGF) or insulin-like growth factor receptors, other interleukins, and so on. Although diphtheria toxin has proved to be effective and relatively nontoxic, other toxins have also been linked to receptor-binding ligands. The trick with these approaches is to find tumors that selectively express receptors and to get the fusion toxin to the tumor. The other trick is to kill all the cells, otherwise clonal populations of the remaining cells will emerge.

## DEATH GENES AND CANCER

Another target for gene therapy has been the programmed cell death or apoptotic pathway that is discussed in Chapter 3. Figure 7–17 illustrates the various pathways involved in apoptosis. A number of different signals have been shown to initiate the apoptosis pathway. As noted in Chapter 3, some

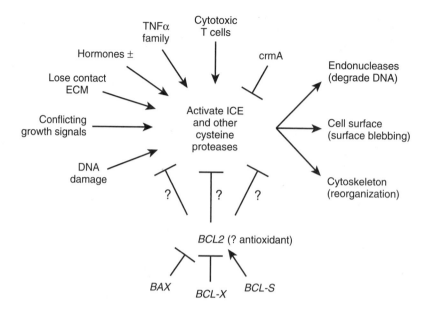

FIGURE 7–17. **The Apoptosis Pathway; Positive and Negative Signals in Programmed Cell Death.** On the left are signals that initiate programmed cell death by activating cysteine proteases. The *Bcl-2* antiapoptosis pathway is depicted in the middle. (See text for explanation.)

of these are involved in normal development; others occur as a result of disease processes, DNA damage, or alterations in cell cycle machinery that produce conflicting proliferation signals. These signals tend to be mediated by *P53*, which is absent or mutated in a large number of tumors. In all these settings, a family of cysteine proteases are induced that lead to degradation of DNA and the structural features of apoptosis. The best studied cysteine protease is interleukin-1β–converting enzyme, which is a mammalian homolog of one of the *C. elegans* genes responsible for the programmed cell death during worm development. There is another family of genes related to *BCL-2*, which serves to modify the apoptosis pathway. *BCL-2* may act as a mitochondrial antioxidant, preventing interleukin-1β–converting enzyme family–induced apoptosis. These molecules act as heterodimers; depending on the partner they may foster *(BAX/BAX)* or prevent *(BCL-2/BCL-2)* cell death. These molecules cannot initiate cell death; rather they serve to modify or regulate the event. Chemotherapy-induced cell death is blocked when *BCL-2* is transfected into malignant cells and high levels of *BCL-2* have been found in a number of malignant cells that are resistant to chemotherapy or radiation treatment.

It is not surprising that the apoptosis area has become an active area of cancer research. The goals have been to induce apoptosis with cytotoxic agents, to enhance the susceptibility of cancer cells to apoptosis or to boost the resistance of normal cells to apoptosis so that large doses of drugs that induce apoptosis can be used to kill cancer cells. Examples have included intravenous infusions of a liposome-p53 complex in mice bearing a malignant breast cancer cell line, hormone therapy of breast and prostate cancer, and decreasing *BCL-2* levels with *BCL-2* antisense (see later).

## DOWNREGULATING ONCOGENES: *myc, mad,* AND *max*

One of the consequences of oncogene overexpression is that oncogenes become a unique target for antitumor therapy because normal cells do not express the oncogene at high levels. If the oncogene is a receptor, as is the case with the EGF receptor family, one might target an antibody to the receptor, blocking the ability of this receptor to transmit cell growth signals. This type of approach has been used in a transgenic mouse model of mammary tumors, produced by overexpression of an EGF-receptor family member. Blocking antibodies—that is, antibodies that bind the receptor but do not induce a growth factor signal—decreased the incidence of tumors by half.

Another oncogene that is involved in many lung cancers is MYC. MYC is a transcription factor that regulates expression of cell proliferation–related genes in early $G_1$. It acts as a heterodimer, forming a complex with another protein called MAX to bind to DNA. A protein that can displace MAX and dimerize with MYC, interfering with its ability to drive expression of $G_1$ genes, is called MAD. Thus MAD antagonizes the effect of MYC on the cell cycle (Fig. 7–18). Recent studies have shown that transfecting tumors with an adenoviral construct that overexpressed MAD slowed the growth of astrocytoma tumor cells that overexpressed MYC and interfered with the ability of these cells to form tumors when injected into other animals. Thus, constitutive expression of oncogenes in cancer cells can be turned off in a number of ways (see discussion of antisense further on), including overexpression of proteins that affect the transcriptional activity of the oncogene. The MYC/MAD/MAX story sounds very much like the regulation of activity of the BCL-2/BAX/BCL-5 apoptosis rescue gene depicted in Figure 7–15.

## MAKING SENSE OF ANTISENSE

The year 1992 was the year of antisense technology, runner-up for *Science*'s Molecule of the Year. It was the molecular biologic designer drug that was to be the cure for cancer. A brief few years later, an enormous number of questions have arisen about how and even if antisense works. Despite the

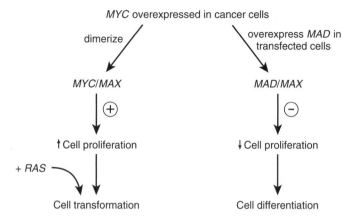

FIGURE 7–18. **Eliminating Oncogene Signals: The** *myc/max/mad* **Story.** To increase cell proliferation, MYC dimerizes with a similar protein, MAX. In the presence of a mutation in another oncogene, such as *ras*, cell transformation occurs. Another partner MAD, can replace MYC, dimerizing with MAX, resulting in decreased proliferation and actual cell differentiation.

fact that several human trials of antisense are in progress, there is increasing concern in the scientific community that this approach to interfering in a precise fashion with expression of a single gene may not be as specific and precise as originally thought.

What is antisense and how is it supposed to work? Figure 7–19 shows that a synthetic oligonucleotide could bind by base pair complementarity to DNA, creating a triple helix that cannot be transcribed, or it could bind to RNA, preventing translation of encoded protein. These oligonucleotides could be delivered to cells and could theretically shut down production of an oncogene. Over time it has become clear that the synthetic oligonucleotides must be short (less than 20 base pairs) and must be phosphothioates rather than phosphodiesters. This involves substituting sulfur for phosphorus in the nucleotides to create a molecule that is more stable and is not degraded by natural cell nucleases. Antisense strategy has been used in a number of experimental settings with dramatic results. However, it does not always work, and conditions must be carefully controlled to ensure that the effects result from specific binding to RNA or DNA. Even with these provisos, there remains considerable controversy about how specific the action of antisense is. The phosphothioates may bind via charge to a number of heparin-binding proteins such as growth factors to induce their effect in a nonantisense fashion and may bind in a nonspecific fashion to induce immune-modulating molecules. The field remains one of active investigation and financial invest-ment by the biotechnology industry. Although the effects that have been observed appear real, the question remains of how these artificial oligonucleo-tides really work.

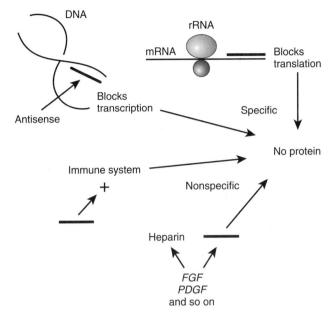

FIGURE 7–19. **Making Sense of Antisense.** An antisense oligonucleotide (bold line) is produced so that it is complementary to the sense strand of the gene of interest. The antisense oligonucleotide either binds to DNA, forming a triple helix, or to mRNA, blocking transcription or translation. Other specific and nonspecific antisense targets have been identified (see text), but the end result is that the antisense oligonucleotide blocks or decreases production of the protein of interest.

## SUGGESTED READING

### General Concepts

Bishop JM: Cancer: The rise of the genetic paradigm. Genes Dev 9:1309–1315, 1995.

Bishop JM: Molecular themes in oncogenesis. Cell 64:235–248, 1991.

Cavenee WK, White RL: The genetic basis of cancer. Sci Am March:72–79, 1995.

Karp JE, Broder S: Molecular foundations of cancer: New targets for intervention. Nat Med 4:309–320, 1995.

### Cell Cycle

Grana X, Reddy EP: Cell cycle control in mammalian cells. Oncogene 11:211–219, 1995.

Merlo A, Herman JG, Mao L, et al: 5′ CpG island methylation is associated with transcriptional silencing of the tumour suppressor p16/CDKN2/MTS1 in human cancers. Nat Med 1:686–692, 1995. [accompanying editorial]

Weinburg RA: The retinoblastoma protein and cell cycle control. Cell 81:323–330, 1995.

### Mismatch Repair

Griffen S: DNA damage, DNA repair and disease. Curr Biol 6:497–499, 1996.

Kolodner R: Mismatch repair: Mechanisms and relationship to cancer susceptibility. Trends in Biochemical Sciences 10:397–401, 1995.

Koshland DE Jr: Molecule of the year: The DNA repair enzyme. Science 266:1925, 1994. [accompanying review and original articles]

Mao L, Lee DJ, Tockman MS, et al: Microsatellite alterations as clonal markers for the detection of human cancer. Proc Natl Acad Sci USA 91:9871–9875, 1994.

### Cancer Gene Therapy

Chen J, Willingham T, Margraf LR, et al: Effects of the MYC oncogene antagonist, MAD, on proliferation, cell cycling and the malignant phenotype of human brain tumor cells. Nat Med 1:638–643, 1995. [accompanying editorial]

Hwang HC, Smythe WR, Elshami AA, et al: Gene therapy using adenovirus carrying the herpes simplex–thymidine kinase gene to treat in vivo models of human malignant mesothelioma and lung cancer. Am J Respir Cell Mol Biol 13:7–16, 1995.

McDonnell TJ, Marn RE, Robertson LE: Implications of apoptotic cell death regulation in cancer therapy. Cancer Biol 6:53–60, 1995.

Murphy JR, vanderSpek JC: Targeting diphtheria toxin to growth factor receptors. Semin Cancer Biol 6:259–267, 1995.

Whartenby KA, Abboud CN, Marrogi AJ, et al: The biology of cancer gene therapy. Lab Invest 72:131–142, 1995.

### Multiple Hit Progression of Cancer

Bodner W, Bishop T, Karran P: Genetic steps in colorectal cancer. Nat Genet 6:217–219, 1994.

Hung J, Kishimoto Y, Sugio K, et al: Allele-specific chromosome 3p deletions occur at an early stage in the pathogenesis of lung carcinoma. JAMA 273:558–563, 1995.

Sugio K, Kishimoto Y, Virmani AK, et al: K-RAS mutations are a relatively late event in the pathogenesis of lung carcinomas. Can Res 54:5811–5815, 1994.

Vogelstein B, Kinzler KW: The multistep nature of cancer. Trends in Genetic Sciences 9:138–141, 1993.

# 8

# Developmental Biology: How Does the Lung Get That Way?

master genes • transcription factors • pattern formation • gel shift assay • DNase footprint • in situ hybridization • protein-protein interactions • zebrafish

Why does the lung form airways and alveoli and put them where they function in the most efficient way? What regulates the cell differentiation that results in type 2 cells being in alveoli and ciliated and mucus-secreting cells being located in large airways? Why is cartilage around large airways only, and what determines where, when, and how much airway smooth muscle forms in the lung? What regulates the expression of surfactant protein genes in type 2 cells and why are they not expressed in type 1 cells? Why is *SPA* and *SPB* expressed in Clara and type 2 cells, but *SPC* is expressed only in type 2 cells? The real answer to these and many other questions about lung development is that no one knows. However, the approaches to these questions and the molecular biologic techniques that have been used to explore development have been one of the most fascinating and rapidly moving areas of science. Of great interest is the fact that developmental and cancer biologists are now talking the same language: regulation of cell proliferation and cell differentiation. Both are asking whether cancer represents a return to the undifferentiated state of cells in the embryo and whether lessons learned from the regulation of development can be applied to understanding and ultimately treating cancer.

Work on the genes that regulate pattern in the fruit fly (*Drosophila*) won a Nobel Prize, and an incredible picture of a fly with eyes on its thighs and elsewhere, appeared on the cover of *Science*. This work defined the "master gene" that converts cells elsewhere in the body into cells that form eyes. One of the great advantages that developmental biologists who study the fly have is the rapid generation time and wide number of cataloged mutations that exist in *Drosophila*. Many of these mutations have been traced to a single gene, so the molecular cause of an anatomic abnormality can be determined. Flies with misplaced antennae, wings, and legs have provided information about genes that determine body pattern, and one of the surprising principles has been that these patterning genes and other genes guiding development are conserved across species: fly, worm, mouse, and human developmental regulators are highly homologous.

## Concept of a Master Gene: Producing an Eye on the Thigh

Many years ago, a mutated gene called eyeless (*ey*) had been described in flies that had deformed or absent eyes. Several years ago a homologous gene called small eye (*sey*) was found in mice and a similar gene called aniridia was found in humans (Fig. 8–1). Mutations in both alleles of *sey* result in mice without eyes. It came as a great surprise that similar genes are involved in eyes as different in structure as that of the fly and the mouse. A team of developmental biologists in Switzerland cloned the mouse *sey* gene and transfected it into *Drosophila* cells that were destined to become parts of other body tissues. To everyone's amazement, flies were born with eyes in every imaginable place: on legs, antennae, wings, and so on. Furthermore, the eyes were structurally normal, with photoreceptor cells that responded to light. It is not clear what role *ey* or *sey* actually plays, how they tell a cell or a tissue to form an eye. However, *ey* and *sey* are certain to be transcription factors that control expression of a number of other genes that are downstream, that is, are expressed only after *ey* or *sey* is first expressed during development of the eye. Thus, all the genes that are responsible for the various structural and signal-transducing functions of the eye, an estimated 2500 genes, depend on the presence of *ey*. Since *ey* actually transforms cells destined to become legs or wings into eyes, it acts as a true master gene. Before one can understand the experiments that resulted in eyes on thighs (and elsewhere), it is necessary to take a small diversion to discuss transcription factors and the roles that they play in regulating gene expression.

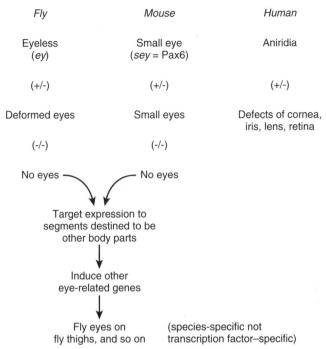

FIGURE 8–1. **An Eye on the Thigh of a Fly.** Fly *ey*, mouse *sey* (which is equivalent to the homeodomain protein Pax-6), and human aniridia are homologous genes. In each, when one allele is lost or mutated [ +/− ], defects in eye development occur. In the fly and mouse, deletion of both alleles has been associated with the absence of eyes. In the experiments described, the mouse *sey* gene was targeted to other body segments of the fly with the resultant appearance of seemingly complete fly eyes on thighs and elsewhere.

# Transcription Factors and Their Families

As discussed in Chapter 1, the initiation of transcription depends on proteins, called transcription factors, that bind to DNA. Only a small portion of the total genetic repertoire is expressed (transcribed) in individual cells at any one time. Most genes in higher organisms are silent. Binding of transcription factors to regulatory portions of DNA or to other transcription factors acts to turn genes on or off. Cell-specific gene expression depends on the right combination of transcription factors being present in a cell at the right time and in the right place. It is these factors that in large part determine whether a specific lung epithelial cell expresses genes as diverse in structure and function as the surfactant proteins, mucus, and cilia. There are relatively few transcription factors, given the tremendous number of cell-specific genes in the body. However, transcription factors work in combination so that more than one is necessary for a cell to express a specific gene, and these combinations of transcription factors interacting with the basal transcription complex provides an almost infinite potential for cell-specific gene transcription.

One important group of transcription factors assembles at the transcription complex, which is most often located within 50 to 150 bases of the transcription initiation site (Fig. 8–2; see also Fig. 1–5). This basal transcription complex, often identified by a TATA nucleotide sequence called the TATA box, serves as a binding site for RNA polymerase, which is essential for transcribing the DNA base code into RNA. Other transcription factor proteins bind elsewhere to DNA, most often 5′ to the promoter, although they may even bind to introns that are 3′ to the promoter. These transcription factors serve to enhance or silence the promoter, resulting in increased or decreased gene transcription. Transcription factors recognize specific segments of DNA or other transcription factors that have bound to DNA and, as a result of their binding, change the conformation of DNA, making it easier or more difficult for the promoter-based transcription complex to initiate transcription of DNA into RNA.

A number of families of transcription factors have been described; their grouping into families is in part determined by the DNA sequence to which they bind and in part relates to the tertiary structure (or motif) of these proteins (Fig. 8–3; see also Fig. 5–1 for discussion of protein structure). One of the first classes of transcription factors to be described was the homeodomain proteins. These proteins have a conserved homeobox, a sequence of 60 amino acids, and they form a tertiary helix-turn-helix structure. The largest group of homeodomain proteins is the *Hox* gene family, which was found to

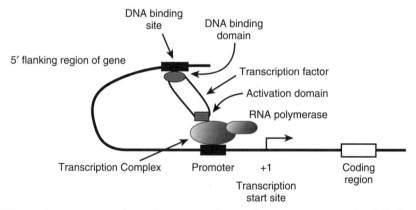

FIGURE 8–2. **Transcription Machinery: Regulation of Gene Expression.** The 5′ flanking region of genes contains a promoter region that is usually close to the transcription start site. The basal transcription machinery assembles here. This multiprotein complex serves as an anchoring site for RNA polymerase, which is the key enzyme required for transcribing DNA into RNA. Enhancers and silencers (rectangle on DNA) consist of specific nucleotide sequences that serve as attachment sites for binding of transcription factors. Transcription factors have a DNA binding domain and a *trans*-activating domain. The latter can link to proteins of the transcription complex, altering the shape of DNA to enhance or silence gene transcription. One transcription factor will often bind to another so that one supplies the DNA binding site and the other the *trans*-activating site.

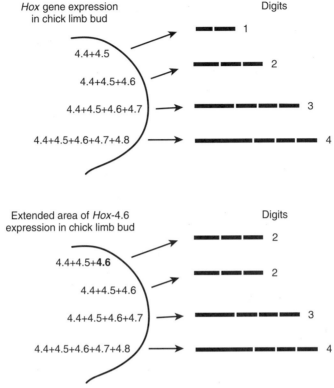

FIGURE 8–3. *Hox* **Genes Provide a Regional "Address" That Specifies Formation of Body Parts.** In the chick limb bud, *Hox* genes 4.4, 4.5, and so on are expressed in overlapping domains so that each area of the developing limb bud expresses a specific set of Hox proteins. Some, such as 4.4, are expressed everywhere; others, such as 4.8, appear only at restricted sites. In the normal chick limb, digit 1 appears at sites 4.4 + 4.5; digit 2 at site 4.4 + 4.5 + 4.6, and so on. If *Hox* 4.6 is misexpressed so that site 4.4 + 4.5 now has the address 4.4 + 4.5 + 4.6, digit 2 (bold) will form instead of digit 1. Similar experiments have shown that the *Hox* "address" is important in rib, vertebrae, and brain morphogenesis.

convey information about body segments in developing *Drosophila*; in essence determining where the wing, leg, and antennae should be placed. These proteins play similar roles in mammals. The *Hox* genes are expressed in overlapping domains, thereby producing a *"Hox* address" that specifies what structure will form at that address (Fig. 8–4). Changing the *Hox* address changes the positioning of major body structures. The downstream genes that the Hox proteins regulate are just being defined, so a complete picture of how they work is not yet available. *Hox* genes are expressed in the developing lung in a pattern that carries information about position and time, suggesting that they may be involved in the patterning of the lung as they are in the patterning of extremities, vertebrae, brain, and so on. Other members of the homeodomain transcription family are TTF1 (about which we will hear more

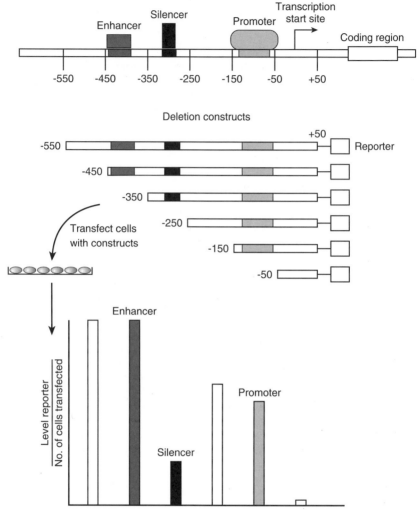

FIGURE 8–4. **Finding Transcriptional Regulatory Regions in Genomic DNA.** The 5′ flanking region of a gene contains a number of specific nucleotide sequences that serve as recognition sites for modulators of gene expression. One can determine where these sequences are by cloning the DNA, linking the DNA to a reporter gene, and creating, with restriction enzymes, deletion constructs that progressively shorten the piece of 5′ flanking DNA. As the DNA is shortened, regulatory sequences are eliminated. This figure depicts regular 100-base pair deletions, but in practice, the size of deletions is determined by convenient restriction enzyme sites. Each construct is then transfected into a cell that expresses the gene of interest, and the level of reporter protein expression, corrected for transcriptional efficiency, is calculated. When an enhancer is deleted (the third construct removes an enhancer between bases −450 and −350), expression of the reporter gene falls. When a silencer is deleted (the fourth construct removes a silencer between −350 and −250), reporter activity increases. The basal promoter is demonstrated between bases −150 and −50. This process defines where major regulators of gene expression lie but does not provide information about the transcription factors that bind to these areas. However, by knowing the base pair sequences in the deleted areas, one can determine if they contain sequences to which specific transcription factors are known to bind.

later and which itself is regulated by a *Hox* gene), the POU domain proteins, and the Pax proteins.

Other important transcription factors are the helix-loop-helix proteins (e.g., myc) and the helix-winged-helix family, whose members include the family of hepatic nuclear factors (HNFs). The HNFs were first described as being important in regulating transcription of liver-specific genes such as albumen, but it was later realized that they control expression of genes in many other tissues, including the lung (see later). Additional important transcription factor families include the steroid hormone superfamily, with zinc finger motifs. Members include the glucocorticoid and thyroid hormone receptors, the retinoid receptors, and the vitamin D receptors; also included are several so-called orphan receptors that have no known ligands. This family of transcription factors tends to act as dimers, either homodimers or heterodimers, forming complexes with themselves or other members of the steroid hormone superfamily. Thus different members of the family have the potential of interacting in order to regulate gene expression. The leucine family of transcription factors include fos and jun and AP1, which can act as proto-oncogenes. The myc protein is a combination of a helix-turn-helix and leucine zipper protein and have been implicated in lung branching morphogenesis.

## Studying Transcriptional Regulation of Gene Expression

Transcription factors have the potential of regulating a wide variety of genes that are associated with development and differentiation. They provide a mechanism for the regulation of gene expression in specific cells or at a specific time that defines the developmental process. How is the process of gene regulation studied? How does one determine what transcription factors are responsible for expression of a specific gene and to what portion of DNA they bind? The answers to these questions allow a discussion of deletion analysis, gel shift assays, DNA footprints, and yeast two-hybrid systems that are used to study protein-protein interactions. The latter step returns the discussion to the amazing "fly on the thigh" story, since the yeast system for studying protein-protein interactions is what was used to prove that *ey* was the master gene of the eye in *Drosophila*.

In order to define regulatory regions of a gene, one must have cloned and sequenced a portion of the 5' flanking region; the genomic DNA upstream from the transcription start site. With sequence in hand, one can search gene data banks to find transcription factors that bind to specific base pair sequences in the 5' flanking region of a gene. However, having the right sequence does not prove that transcription factor binding to that sequence actually occurs. To do this, the piece of genomic DNA together with a vector containing a reporter gene and a cell line that expresses or can be induced to express the gene being studied are all that one needs. The vector containing the 5′ flanking region and the reporter gene is transfected into the cell line, the nuclear proteins of the cell bind to the DNA, and transcription of the DNA creates a signal from the reporter (see Fig. 8–4). The amount of the signal is proportional to the activity of the nuclear transcription factors in the cell and to the potential of the transfected piece of DNA to be activated by those factors. This type of measurement requires only transient transfection of the cell. The 5′ flanking region is then systematically shortened by cutting it with restriction enzymes, creating deletion mutants that are again transfected into the cell; the degree of reporter activity is then measured. The changes that occur in reporter gene activity reflect the deletion of enhancer and silencer elements in the regulatory region of the gene.

In order to prove that a nuclear protein is binding in a specific fashion to that portion of DNA, a gel shift assay is performed. A specific portion of the 5′ flanking region is labeled with a radioisotope and exposed to nuclear extract of the cell expressing that gene. If nuclear proteins bind to that piece of DNA, they retard its migration in a nondenaturing gel (Fig. 8–5). Thus, labeled DNA that is free of protein migrates rapidly in the gel, and DNA to

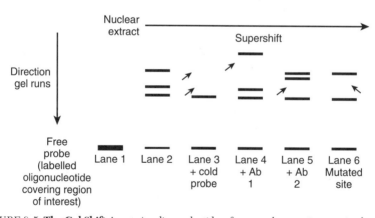

FIGURE 8–5. **The Gel Shift Assay.** An oligonucleotide—for example, covering a region between −45 and −350 in Figure 8–4—is made and labeled. The probe, free of any nuclear extract, is loaded on a gel and runs to the bottom of the gel (*Lane 1*). *Lane 2* through *Lane 6* have nuclear extracts from cells expressing the gene of interest mixed with the labeled probes. Since these cells contain transcription factors that are involved in regulating expression of the gene, the transcription factors bind to the appropriate bases of the oligonucleotide, retarding its migration in the gel. By adding an excess of unlabeled probe, one can separate specific protein-DNA interactions (*arrows* in *Lane 3*) from nonspecific nuclear protein DNA interactions. If one adds antibodies to transcription factors suspected to be involved in DNA binding, the specific antibody will bind to the DNA-protein complex, further retarding its migration in the gel. Since more than one transcription factor can bind to the DNA sequence of the probe, or the bands may represent DNA-protein-protein complexes, a second antibody may identify a second relevant nuclear transcription factor. One can also determine which nucleotides are important for DNA-protein interactions by mutating sequences of the DNA probe and changing bands in the gel retardation assay as in *Lane 6*.

which nuclear proteins have bound migrates less rapidly. A gel with nuclear extract from a cell not expressing the gene being studied or DNA without nuclear extract added is run as a control. The specificity of the binding can be tested by showing that cold (unlabeled) oligonucleotides compete off the slowly migrating band. If a specific transcription factor is suspected, an antibody can be added to the mixture, and the band with DNA and nuclear protein will be supershifted because the addition of an antibody to the protein will produce a complex that migrates even more slowly in the gel. Labeled nucleotides with mutated binding sites can also be used to identify the portion of DNA to which proteins have bound.

Another way to determine the specific bases to which the protein has bound is to expose a radiolabeled DNA–nuclear protein complex to degradation with DNase. This enzyme digests bases without bound protein but cannot digest protein-DNA complexes. The result is a picture similar to that seen in Figure 8–6. A lane without nuclear protein can be run as a control, and the identity of the bases binding to protein can be read. Finally, the DNA can be mutated in order to determine the exact bases that are important in the interaction. If no protein has been previously described that binds to that sequence of bases, the transcription factor protein can be isolated by running the nuclear extract over a column that contains the DNA to which it binds. After other proteins run through the column, the DNA-binding protein can be eluted and sequenced.

These are all in vitro studies performed under highly artificial circumstances and may be subject to experimental artifact. The only way to determine if a specific piece of DNA truly confers cell or tissue specificity in life is to make transgenic mice with the important elements of the 5′ flanking region driving a reporter gene. The transgenic mouse will then express the reporter gene in those tissues or cells with transcription factors that bind to the DNA and drive transcription of the reporter. Studies such as this have shown that the first 3.7-kb of the SPC regulatory region are sufficient to limit expression of the reporter to the lung and to Clara and type 2 cells within the lung. However, an additional 20 kb are needed before SPC is expressed only in type 2 cells, as is the endogenous gene. Similar study of the Clara cell secretory protein (CCSP) has shown that a short piece of the 5′ flanking region is sufficient to limit expression of a reporter to the correct parts of the airway epithelium, but that a much larger piece is needed to re-create the same expression pattern in time as the endogenous gene. Surprisingly, only a few hundred bases of 5′ flanking region of SPB provide the appropriate information for its organ and cell specificity.

A number of recent studies have characterized some elements of cell-specific gene expression in the lung, but have not fully defined why, for example, SPC is expressed only in type 2 cells of the adult lung. Studies such as these (Fig. 8–7) have shown that some genes, such as SPB, can be regulated by one transcription factor in the Clara cell and another in the type 2 cell, thus providing a mechanism for differential regulation in time in these two

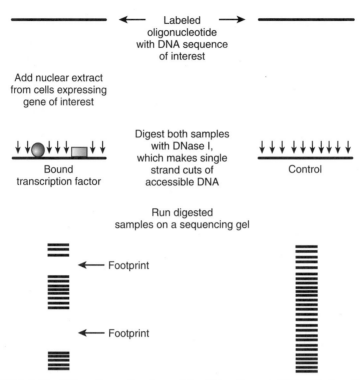

**FIGURE 8–6. The DNase Protection Assay: Identifying Bases to Which Nuclear Proteins Have Bound.** The labeled oligonucleotide probe is either mixed with nuclear extract from cells expressing the gene of interest or is free of nuclear extract (control). The probes are then exposed to DNase I, which cuts all exposed DNA single strands at each nucleotide. The resultant mixtures are then separated in a gel. The DNA probe that is free of nuclear extract separates into a series of individual bases. The DNA to which transcription factors have bound is protected from cutting by DNase and is not cut at those places where protein-DNA complexes were present, leaving behind footprints whose nucleic acids can be identified by prior knowledge of the probe sequence. The specificity of the footprint can be determined by similar studies with oligonucleotides in which specific bases have been changed. It is possible that more than one protein has bound to the footprinted areas.

*SPB*-expressing cells. They have also shown that a transcription factor can act as a silencer for one gene but an enhancer for another gene. In addition, a transcription factor can act to induce more than one gene, as is the case with TTF1, which activates several of the surfactant proteins, the CCSP, as well as thyroid-specific genes. Although TTF1 appears to be an important transcription factor for all the surfactant genes, it also serves an important morphogenic function because in its absence, lung branching does not occur. HNFs are also extensively involved in regulating expression of the surfactant proteins and CCSP. They also serve important morphogenic functions, since knockouts of HNF3β result in embryonic lethality.

One transcription factor can regulate many genes

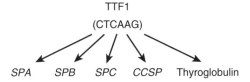

One gene can be regulated by many transcription factors

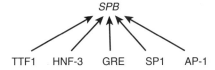

One DNA element can be regulated by two different transcription factors

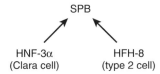

FIGURE 8–7. **Transcription Factors and Lung Genes.** TTF1, originally described as the transcription factor responsible for regulating thyroid-specific genes including thyroglobulin (tyroglob), has been shown to be an important regulator of a number of lung epithelial cell genes. The (CTCAAG) nucleotide sequence defines a DNA binding element common to all the genes. The middle panel in the figure makes the point that most genes are regulated by a number of transcription factors, each with their own unique DNA binding sites. The bottom panel shows that the same general area of DNA contains binding sites that provide a mechanism for independent Clara cell and type 2 cell upregulate expression of the *SPB* gene. The type 2 cell produces HFH-8, which binds to this region, whereas the Clara cell produces HNF-3α, which also binds to this site. Thus, the two cells can regulate *SPB* expression independently, allowing different timing of expression.

# When and Where Genes Are Expressed: In Situ Hybridization

Northern blots and polymerase chain reaction measure the presence of an mRNA for a specific gene. Neither of these methods provides information about which of the many cells in a developing organ actually express the gene. Scientists who study lung development have found that the surfactant protein genes for *SPA* and *SPB* are expressed in both Clara and type 2 cells, whereas the *SPC* gene is expressed only in type 2 cells. The observations were made by using a histologic Northern blot called in situ hybridization (Fig. 8–8). This method demonstrates the exact cells that express a specific mRNA. To do this, a labeled antisense RNA probe is hybridized to the sense mRNA expressed in tissue sections, which are on a slide. The principle of

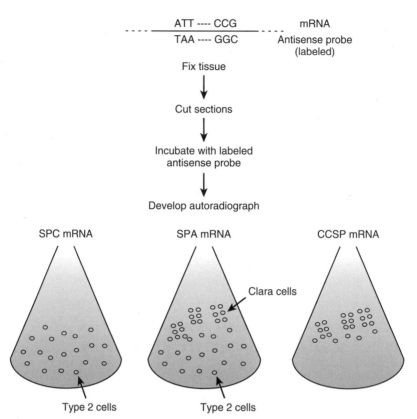

FIGURE 8–8. **Where Genes are Expressed: In Situ Hybridization.** To localize sites of mRNA expression, an antisense probe to a unique portion of the mRNA of interest is labeled. Although sulfur-35 is the isotope most often used, nonradioactive methods are gaining popularity. Tissue is fixed and sections prepared, with special attention being paid to preventing RNA degradation. The sections are incubated with the labeled probe and developed. The diagrams at the bottom depict the sites of *SPC* expression (only type 2 cells), *SPA* expression (type 2 cells and Clara cells), and CCSP expression (Clara cells).

complementarity and hybridization at a known level of stringency is the same as with a Northern blot except that the mRNA being measured is in cells within a section of tissue instead of on a filter. The trick is to fix the tissues so that the RNA is preserved in a form that will hybridize to the antisense probe. To ensure that the signal, which most often is radioactive particles, is specific for the RNA, control sections are hybridized with sense probes that should not hybridize because they are not complementary. Studies such as these have, in addition to the cellular patterns of surfactant protein gene expression noted earlier, characterized the developmentally regulated sites of expression of a number of genes in the lung. They have shown that *SPC* and a type 1 cell gene called *T1α* are expressed in the same cells of the earliest lung bud, but that their expression diverges early in development. This observation of early expression of two genes that mark the two cells of the fully differentiated alveolar epithelium is puzzling. It seems unlikely that type 1 and type 2 cells exist from the time that the primitive lung bud first forms; rather, the genes must serve some as yet undetermined function during early development that in the mature lung lies in the two different cell types.

## Turning Genes off During Development

There are now a number of genes in the developing lung that are initially expressed in many cells and later in development are restricted to one or a few specific cells. It is most likely that these genes serve some function during early development that is no longer required by the cells as the lung matures. One might expect that proliferation-related genes, motility genes, and cell adhesion and ion transport genes fall into this category. *T1α*, the type 1 cell gene mentioned previously, is expressed in much of the epithelium of the developing lung, but only in type 1 cells of the mature lung. It is also expressed in virtually all neuronal structures in early development but is rapidly downregulated (turned off) in all neuronal tissue except the choroid plexus.

Regardless of function, how does a cell go about turning off a gene that is no longer needed? Figure 8–9 illustrates a number of different possibilities related to competing transcription factors. Chapter 7 has already introduced DNA methylation, a mechanism that appears to be important in development. As discussed in Chapter 7, methylation of CpG islands in 5′ flanking regions of DNA make these sites inaccessible to DNA-binding transcription factors and is one reason that the growth suppression gene *P16* is not expressed in some tumors. Since transcription factors cannot bind to DNA, the gene is not transcribed. Selective DNA methylation can be regulated on a cell by cell basis by an enzyme called maintainance methylase; when the enzyme is expressed, CpG islands are methylated and genes are not expressed; when methylase is turned off, gene expression occurs.

Methylation has also been shown to be responsible for the interesting phenomenon of genomic imprinting. In this instance, in contrast to most genes that express maternal and paternal allelles, one parent provides the only allelle. This is the case with the *IGF2* gene, which is inherited from the father only and the *IGF2* receptor gene, which is inherited from the mother only. It appears that the maternal copy of the *IGF2* gene is methylated and therefore is not transcribed, whereas the paternal copy is methylated for the receptor gene. The molecular and teleologic reason for this imprinting is not yet clear.

## Growth Factors Are Important: Dominant Negative Mutants

Despite the previously discussed focus on transcription factors, there are many other molecules involved in and regulating the developmental process.

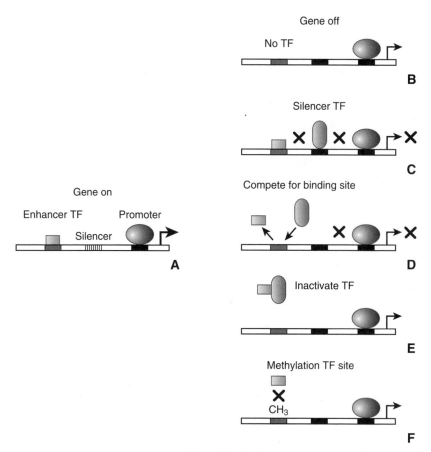

FIGURE 8–9. **How to Turn a Gene Off.** *A,* The diagram shows the 5′ flanking region of a gene, the promoter in black, a silencer element *(striped)* and an enhancer element that is cross-hatched. When the gene is on, that is, being transcribed *(thick arrow),* the basal transcriptional machinery is in place and a transcription factor *(TF)* binds to the enhancer element. The gene can be turned off (inactivated) by a number of different mechanisms. *B,* There is no enhancer–transcription factor being produced by the cell. Transcription might occur at a very low level dictated by the promoter. In this case, developmental expression of a cell-specific gene is determined by production of the transcription factor. *C,* A transcription factor binds to the silencer element. It may either block activation by the enhancer element, allowing low levels of transcription to occur, or it may act on the promoter to inactivate the basal transcriptional process. *D,* The silencer transcription factor competes with the enhancer transcription factor for the enhancer site. *E,* A protein binds to the enhancer transcription factor and prevents its activation of the enhancer element. *F,* Methylation of CpG-rich areas of the enhancer prevent access to the enhancer site.

Matrix proteins, cell adhesion molecules, and growth factors have all been implicated in the deveopment of the lung. The fibroblast growth factor (FGF) family of genes has proved critical in the development of the limb and more recently in the development of the lung. One of the most effective ways of determining the importance of a gene in development is to knock it out. This technique has been presented in Chapter 4. However, another way to eliminate the function of a gene or protein is to express another protein that acts to impair the function of the gene of interest. In this approach to interrupting gene function, the mutated gene may produce a transcription factor that binds to DNA but is unable to activate transcription. In binding to the DNA, it competes with the normal transcription factor, which cannot then perform its transcriptional activation (Fig. 8–10). Another example is production of an enzyme that binds substrate but cannot cleave the substrate to activate it. In each instance, the mutant protein, expressed at a high level, competes with the normal protein and completely inhibits its function.

The evidence that FGF plays an important role in lung development comes from several experiments. One of the most interesting, again from the fly, was a mutant fly with no trachea, found to be associated with a mutation in the *Drosophila* FGF receptor. In the fly, this receptor served to transduce signals induced by the FGF that leads to migration of epithelial cells during formation of the fly trachea. Subsequently, another group created a dominant negative form of the FGF receptor, which bound the FGF ligand but did not transduce a signal. The mutant receptor had no cytoplasmic tyrosine kinase signal-transducing domain. The mutant receptor competed with the normal receptor for FGF ligand, forming a complex with the normal receptor to inactivate it. Widespread expression of this mutant would result in embryonic lethality because FGF is required for the formation of many organs. However, using the trick of driving expression of the dominant negative mutant with the *SPC* promoter, limited its effect to the developing lung. This transgenic mouse formed an embryonic lung bud, but no branching of airways occurred, no alveoli formed, and the mice died at birth. Thus, the FGF receptor family of genes plays a crucial but as yet undefined role in lung development.

## The Eye on the Thigh

The preceding discussion has focused on the DNA binding domains of transcription factors. However, it is not the DNA binding region that activates gene transcription; this region determines to which DNA sequence the factor binds. It is the *trans*-activating domain of the transcription factor that is responsible for actually inducing gene expression. This portion of the transcription factor binds to other proteins, usually in the transcription complex itself, to alter DNA configuration and enhance transcription (see Fig. 8–2). A system that uses yeast biochemistry has been developed to define the mechanisms by which enhancers and silencers bind to transcription complex proteins (Fig. 8–11). This system uses the yeast *GAL4* gene activator, which binds to a known upstream DNA sequence and the *GAL4 trans*-activation region, which activates transcription in yeast of an enzyme that converts galactose

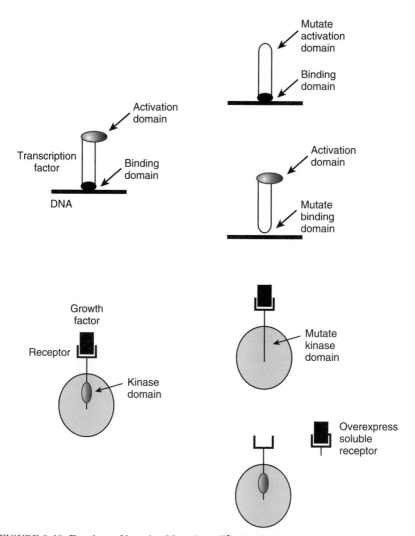

FIGURE 8–10. **Dominant Negative Mutations: Eliminating a Gene or a Receptor.** Genes can be turned off without creating gene knockouts. Dominant negative experiments target mutations that interfere with normal gene function by creating nonfunctional proteins that compete with normal proteins for ligands. In the case of transcription factors, activation or DNA binding domains are mutated so that they are nonfunctional. The mutated gene is then overexpressed in cells or in transgenic mice, competing with the normal protein for its DNA or activation binding site. In the case of a growth factor receptor, the gene is mutated so that the signaling domain is removed or the receptor lacks an anchoring site and is secreted. In each case, the mutant protein competes with the normal receptor protein for ligand, which binds but cannot activate the signaling pathway.

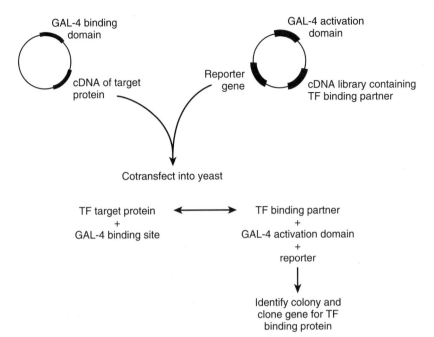

FIGURE 8–11. **Protein-Protein Interactions: The GAL4 Two-Hybrid System.** GAL4 is a transcription factor produced in yeast but not in mammals. It has a DNA binding domain and an activation domain with specific DNA recognition sites for each. Two-hybrid systems allow one to construct two-hybrid proteins that use the GAL4 system fused to other proteins. In this experiment, the hybrid constructs include the transcription factor *(TF)* of interest fused to the GAL4 DNA binding domain, and a cDNA expression library fused to the GAL4 activation domain. The two hybrids are cotransfected into yeast, and following various selection steps the cells that express the transcription factor and its binding partner will activate the reporter gene hooked to the activation domain, thereby identifying cells that contain the binding protein of interest. These cells are isolated, and the binding partner cDNA is cloned and sequenced. In this case, the transcription factor and its partner substituted for GAL4, creating the link between the two GAL4 sites.

to glucose. The details of this method are explained in the legend for Figures 8–11 and 8–12.

A variation of this so-called two-hybrid system is what was used to produce the eye on the thigh experiments that identified the master gene of the eye. In these experiments, discussed at the beginning of this chapter, transgenic flies were created that expressed the GAL4 binding site (actually multiple GAL4 binding sites) hooked to either the fly *ey* gene or the mouse *sey* gene in all cells (see Fig. 8–1). The oocytes of these flies were then transfected with an enhancer trap construct that contained the *GAL4* gene driven by a very weak promoter. This construct integrates randomly in the fly genome. If it inserts behind a strong tissue-specific enhancer and is close to the gene expressing the GAL4 binding sites, it will bind to the GAL4 binding sites and activate the *ey* or the *sey* gene in that tissue, leading to its strong

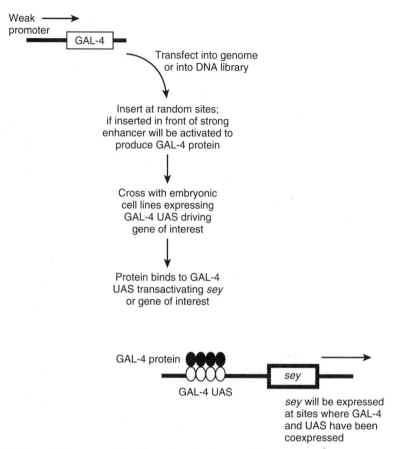

FIGURE 8–12. **The Eye on the Fly on the Thigh: Using the GAL4 System and Enhancer Traps.** The eye on the thigh experiments used a GAL4 cDNA that was driven by a weak promoter. Thus, when transfected into cells, it is not transcribed at a detectable rate. This construct was transfected into fly oocytes inserting at random into the fly genome. When the construct is inserted or trapped behind a strong enhancer (the enhancer trap), the GAL4 is expressed. If cells containing this transcript are crossed with cells expressing the GAL4 upstream activating site driving the *ey* or *sey* gene, those cells expressing both will activate *ey* or *sey* and an eye will form at that site. The process is random, so eyes may form on the thigh, the head, the wing, or elsewhere. The very fact that expression of *ey* or *sey* changes the fate of the cells normally destined to be thigh or wing cells proves that *ey* or *sey* are eye master genes.

expression. When this happens, eyes form and they form in all tissues in which the two hybrids have been expressed. Thus *ey* or *sey* can produce fly eyes, showing that the transcriptional activator is not species-specific but the response to the activator is; that is, both the fly and the mouse transcription factors produce the compound eye of the fly. These experiments now provide a way to determine the sequence of genes that are activated in forming the eye and to examine the evolutionary pathways that led to the formation of mammalian eyes.

It now seems possible that many complex organs have a master gene that is capable of initiating a cascade of events leading to formation of a specific structure. It may take some time to find the master gene of the lung, especially since the fly has no lung to be induced.

## Developmental Biology and the Zebrafish, a Vertebrate Relative

In 1995, the Nobel Prize for Medicine and Physiology was given to Drs. Nusslein-Volhard and Weischaus for their work that showed that cataloging fly *(Drosophila melanogaster)* mutations could reveal genes that are involved in the regulation of development. Many of the genes, such as *eyeless,* have been cloned, their mammalian counterparts identified, and their functions defined. Despite the tremendous impact that fly mutagenesis has had on developmental biology, the fact that the fly is an invertebrate limits to some extent its applicability to humans. In addition to the obvious lack of a notochord, the embryonic backbone, which is involved in the formation of the brain, heart, gut derivatives, vessels, and skin cells, has no correlate in the fly. Enter *Danio rerio,* the zebrafish—a transparent, rapidly generating, externally developing vertebrate; the developmental model system of 1996. The zebrafish has everything mammals have, except that fins substitute for limbs, kidneys are primitive and, unfortunately, there are no lungs. Two groups of investigators, one of which includes Dr. Nusslein-Volhard, have analyzed a total of 1800 mutations representing defects in 500 different genes that produce the structural form and function of the zebrafish.

The approach that was taken to define genes involved in zebrafish development is illustrated in Figure 8–13; it is called saturation mutagenesis. Adult males are fed the chemical mutagen ethyl nitrosourea (ENU in figure) in a concentration that produces approximately one random DNA point mutation per genome. Sperm from the exposed males is used to fertilize donor eggs. One member of the initial progeny of this artificial mating (the F1 generation, which is heterozygous for the mutation) is crossed with another to produce 50% heterozygotes in the F2 generation, and this generation, when crossed, results in 25% homozygotes, which are analyzed for phenotype using the dissecting microscope. Because the embryos are transparent, virtually all gross developmental defects can be identified visually. Once mutations have been identified and reproduced, they can be linked to the increasing number of zebrafish genetic markers that will soon result in a genetic map of the zebrafish, and the gene ultimately can be positionally cloned. Alternatively, libraries of zebrafish chromosomes can be used to rescue the mutant phenotype. Once a large piece of DNA has been shown to correct the defect, it can be successively deleted until a gene is isolated. Analogies to *Drosophila,* mouse, or human DNA can, of course, provide insights into gene structure.

Perhaps not surprising is the fact that a number of mutations have

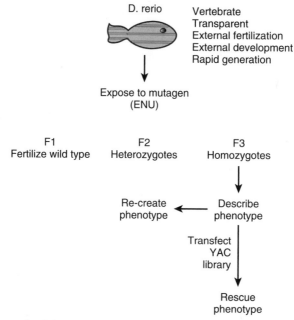

FIGURE 8–13. **Zebrafish: The Newest Tool of Developmental Biologists.** The zebrafish has many features that make it a perfect model for the study of vertebrate development. Its rapid generation, external fertilization, and development make it the vertebrate equivalent of *Drosophila*. Its transparency allows easy characterization of morphologic mutations. The fish are exposed to an external mutagen in a dose calculated to produce approximately one mutation per genome. Sperm are taken from each male and used to generate several generations of families, which lead to a large number of homozygotes, which are then characterized by morphologic phenotype. Some genes will be missed because they are lethal mutants, and some will generate subtle phenotypes that are not recognized. Sperm from homozygotes with specific phenotypes is used to reconfirm the phenotype; genomic libraries of zebrafish can then be used to transfect genes into germ cells to determine what piece of DNA, and therefore what gene, rescues the phenotype.

already been identified that have human counterparts. This is particularly true of heart, central nervous system, and hematopoietic abnormalities. Although much work remains to be done to identify specific genes and their functions in the mutant zebrafish—genes that have been given such wonderfully descriptive names such as heart and soul, santa, bubblehead, mind bomb, and bashful—*Danio rerio* represent a major step forward in the science of developmental biology.

## SUGGESTED READING

### Regulation of Transcription

Cardoso WV: Transcription factors and pattern formation in the developing lung. Am J Physiol 13:L429–L442, 1995.

Morgan BA, Izpisua-Belmonte J, Duboule D, et al: Targeted misexpression of Hox-4.6 in the avian limb bud causes apparent homeotic transformations. Nature 358:236–239, 1992.

Whitsett JA, Korfhagen TR: Regulation of gene transcription in respiratory epithelial cells. Am J Respir Cell Mol Biol 14:118–120, 1996.

### The Eye of the Fly

Halder G, Callaerts P, Gehring WJ: Induction of ectopic eyes by targeted expression of the eyeless gene in *Drosophila.* Science 267:1788–1792, 1995. [accompanying editorial comment]

### Transgenic Models

Glasser SW, Korfhagen TR, Wert S, et al: Transgenic models for the study of pulmonary development and disease. Am J Physiol 267:L489–L497, 1994.

### Dominant Negative Mutations

Peters K, Werner S, Liao X, et al: Targeted expression of a dominant negative FGF receptor blocks branching and epithelial differentiation of the mouse lung. EMBO J 13:3296, 1994.

Sheppard D: Dominant negative mutants: Tools for the study of protein function in vitro and in vivo. Am J Respir Cell Mol Biol 11:1–6, 1994.

### Zebrafish

Driever W, Fishman MC: The zebrafish: Heritable disorders in transparent embryos. J Clin Invest 98(Suppl):S41–S46, 1996.

Holder N, McMahon A: Genes from zebrafish screens. Nature 384:515–516, 1996.

Eisen JS: Zebrafish make a big splash. Cell 87:969–977, 1996.

# Acquired Immunodeficiency Syndrome

retroviruses • HIV-1 vectors • viral dynamics • branched chain DNA assay • DNA microarray—the chip

In the United States, 40,000 persons become infected with the human immunodeficiency virus (HIV) each year. Worldwide there are now 21 million individuals who are infected, 90% of them in the developing world. The scientific progress made in 1996, largely employing the methods of molecular biology, has provided the first real sign of a breakthrough in the battle against acquired immunodeficiency syndrome (AIDS). The importance of this scientific progress was recognized by *Time* magazine, which named an HIV virologist its "Man of the Year." Until recently, AIDS was viewed as an HIV-induced disease following an initial infection that occurred only after a long latent period during which the virus was dormant. Recent molecular studies of viral dynamics have not only redefined the latent period, the course of HIV viremia, and mechanisms of immune cell infection, but also have dictated new approaches to therapy. Investigations of individuals who are not infected despite multiple exposures to HIV, or those with prolonged survival once infected, have helped define a new set of viral coreceptors. Infection-protecting mutations in these receptors have been discovered, and these may be new targets for therapy to prevent infection. The treatment of HIV-infected individuals has been revolutionized by the introduction of protease inhibitors, and new molecular methods are being applied to define protease resistance mutations. These latter techniques hold the promise of introducing a new era of molecular diagnostics for many diseases.

This chapter illustrates the molecular concepts and techniques that have been responsible for these advances. It begins with a discussion of retroviruses and how knowledge of the HIV retrovirus has produced a potential new vector for gene therapy.

## What Are Retroviruses and How Do They Work?

Retroviruses are such effective invaders of cells because they capture the host cell genome and use it to assist in their own propagation and secretion. In the process, they can induce cell tranformation if the retrovirus is oncogenic or result in widespread dissemination if the retrovirus is HIV. Retroviruses have no DNA and thus must use the host cell's replicative machinery for proliferation. The RNA virus invades a cell (see later discussion of HIV receptors) and its RNA is reverse-transcribed into DNA by one of its three genes—a reverse polymerase or transcriptase. If the host cell divides, the viral DNA is then incorporated into the host cell's genome so that each time the cell replicates, the virus does also. Simple retroviruses have only three genes; *pol* (the RNA polymerase), *gag* (a structural packaging protein), and *env* (a viral coat or outer shell protein). Retroviruses also contain a strong promoter with many repeats in it (called the long terminal repeat or LTR) and a strong enhancer. Figure 9–1 shows a typical retrovirus and illustrates how it uses a host cell for its own propagation.

The retroviral vectors, discussed in Chapter 5, have been altered to remove their LTRs and their packaging gene so that even though they have integrated into the host cell genome and will be replicated when host cell DNA is replicated, the retrovirus cannot be packaged and secreted to infect other cells. The HIV virus differs from simple retroviruses in that it contains nine rather than three genes. The six additional genes encode proteins that regulate viral gene expression and account for HIV's ability to kill host cells (Fig. 9–2).

## Using Human Immunodeficiency Virus as a Vector for Gene Therapy

The murine leukemia retroviruses that are routinely used for gene therapy can infect dividing cells only. However, many of the cells one may wish to

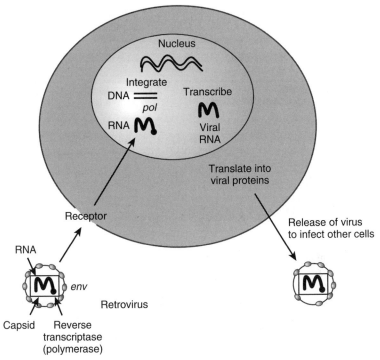

FIGURE 9–1. **How Retroviruses Work.** Typical retroviruses enter cells via receptors that interact with the retroviral env protein. Within the nucleus, the viral RNA is reverse-transcribed into DNA via the reverse transcriptase encoded by the *pol* gene and integrates into the DNA of cells undergoing DNA synthesis. The viral RNA is then transcribed and translated, and the viral protein leaves the cell ready to infect neighboring cells.

target for gene therapy—for example, neuronal cells, hematologic stem cells, hepatocytes, and lung epithelial cells—are not normally dividing. This has been one of the major limitations of retroviruses in human gene therapy. The lentivirus family, of which HIV is a member, is able to infect nondividing cells. Two of the HIV genes depicted in Figure 9–2, *vpr* and *ma* (matrix), interact with the nuclear transport machinery of the cell to help shuttle HIV into the nucleus independent of the state of cell proliferation. A recent article reports that an HIV vector, modified by removal of packaging and LTR portions of the HIV genome, can safely infect nondividing cells (Fig. 9–3). If the HIV *env* gene, which limits its entry to cells of the immune system, is removed and replaced with a viral *env* that allows more promiscuous cell infection, a large number of different types of cells, including neuronal cells, can be efficiently transfected in vivo, independent of their proliferative state. Although much work needs to be done to create efficient viral packaging systems that will produce large quantities of the re-engineered HIV vector,

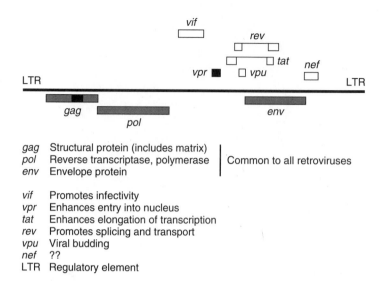

FIGURE 9–2. **The HIV-1 Genome.** HIV-1 contains an extra six genes, which code for proteins that promote infectivity and transcription as well as enhancing nuclear entry (solid black), allowing integration into the DNA of nondividing cells. (See discussion in text of using HIV-1 as a vector.) LTR, long terminal repeat.

and to explore the potential use of lentiviruses other than HIV, this new vector system provides an exciting tool for gene therapists.

## Measuring Virion Load: Branched Chain DNA Amplification

One of the early dogmas of AIDS was that following infection with HIV, the virus was sequestered in lymphoid tissues and was dormant for long periods. Only after a long latent period did the virus activate, kill T cells, and result in the many manifestations of immunodeficiency. Recent studies using new measurements of circulating viral load have provided a dramatically different picture of the course of HIV infection and have, as a result, changed the strategies of drug therapy for AIDS.

Figure 9–4 demonstrates the present view of viremia with HIV that has resulted from these studies. Following the initial infection with HIV and the immune response that it induces, there continues to be a stable level of circulating virus during the period previously thought to represent viral latency. The steady state of viremia results from the balance of viral production, viral death, and T-cell turnover. On average, 10 billion HIV virions are produced each day, with a mean life span of 0.3 days. Infected mononuclear cells have an average life span of 2.2 days. The average HIV generation

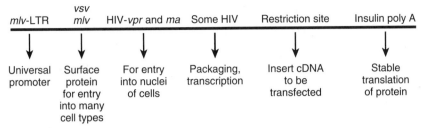

| *mlv*-LTR | *vsv*<br>*mlv* | HIV-*vpr* and *ma* | Some HIV | Restriction site | Insulin poly A |
|-----------|------------|-------------------|----------|------------------|----------------|
| Universal promoter | Surface protein for entry into many cell types | For entry into nuclei of cells | Packaging, transcription | Insert cDNA to be transfected | Stable translation of protein |

FIGURE 9–3. **Redesigning HIV-1 DNA for Use in Gene Therapy.** The vector depicted in this figure takes advantage of the features of several viral genomes. The *mlv* (murine leukemia virus) is a universal promoter. Either *mlv* or *vsv* (vesicular stomatitis virus) env protein is used because it binds to the receptors on many different cells, not just CD4 + cells as does HIV-1. The HIV *vpr* and *ma* genes (see Fig. 9–2) are included to promote nuclear entry and integration into the DNA of nondividing cells. A restriction site is in place so that the cDNA to be transfected can be inserted. The insulin poly A tail provides for stability of the transcribed mRNA. LTR, long terminal repeat.

time—the time from release of HIV viral particles from one cell until they infect and cause viral release from another cell—was 2.6 days. Thus, virus is being made, infecting and killing CD4 + cells at an extremely high rate during the period previously thought to represent "viral latency."

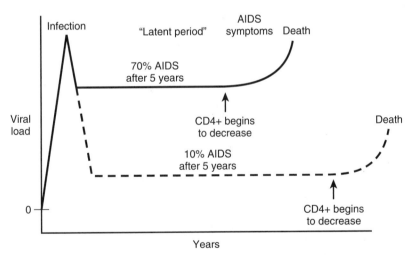

FIGURE 9–4. **The Course of HIV-1 Viremia and Its Relation to Clinical Outcomes.** Viral load is depicted on the vertical axis and time from initial infection is seen on the horizontal axis. Following the initial infection, viral load decreases as a result of the host immune response to HIV-1. Different individuals experience different steady state levels of plasma viremia. This results from the balance of viral replication and cell killing, as discussed in the text. Those individuals with high steady state levels of HIV tend to have short asymptomatic "latent" periods, whereas those with low steady state levels tend to have long asymptomatic periods. At a time when HIV becomes T-trophic, CD4 + counts begin to fall and individuals acquire progressive symptoms of AIDS.

Late in the disease, viral load rises, CD4+ cell counts fall, and clinical symptoms appear. Recent studies have shown that a single measure of virion load is a highly accurate predictor of time from initial infection with HIV to clinically evident AIDS. The virion load assay appears to be a better predictor of time to clinical symptoms than does the CD4+ count. A vivid comparison of the two measures is that viral load is equivalent to the speed of a train approaching a wall, whereas the CD4+ count is equivalent to the distance between the train and the wall. It should be evident that this picture of high levels of HIV production and CD4+ cell killing presents a strong argument for early antiviral therapy.

The test that changed the thinking about HIV dynamics and argued for early rather than late therapy of infected individuals is the branched DNA signal amplification assay, a measure of the plasma level of HIV mRNA. The assay has become so valuable as a predictor of course and assay of response to therapy that it is replacing the CD4+ count and is in the process of generating a $100 million per year biotechnology business. The principle of the branched DNA signal amplification test is illustrated in Figure 9–5. Most of the methods used to assess activity of HIV have been limited by being either indirect (e.g., the CD4+ cell count) or insensitive. Polymerase chain reaction (PCR) for HIV mRNA in plasma has been used; however, as discussed in Chapter 2, PCR measurements are not quantitative. The branched DNA test (see Fig. 9–5) captures HIV mRNA, which hybridizes to oligonucleotides that are designed to bind to the *pol* sequence of HIV. These oligonucleotides have an overhang sequence that binds to oligonucleotides coated on the surface of a microtiter plate. A second oligonucleotide, which binds to additional overhang sequences, is added to this dimerized mix. This target probe has a series of 15 branches, each of which contains sequences complementary to an alkaline phosphatase probe. It is this probe that amplifies the RNA signal; the amplification is not of the RNA as in the PCR method but of the colorimetric readout of captured HIV RNA. For the test, viral particles are removed from a sample of plasma, RNA is extracted, and the prepackaged reaction is run, comparing the readout to a standard curve.

# Human Immunodeficiency Virus Coreceptors: Exposed but Uninfected—Sexually Promiscuous but Virus-Free

It has been known for years that HIV infects cells that express CD4 because the HIV envelope protein (gp120) binds to the CD4 receptor. However, the CD4 receptor alone is not sufficient for HIV binding to and infection of immune system cells. Further, it has been known that HIV isolates from newly infected individuals could bind and gain entry into macrophages and T lymphocytes but not T-cell lines that had been in culture for long periods.

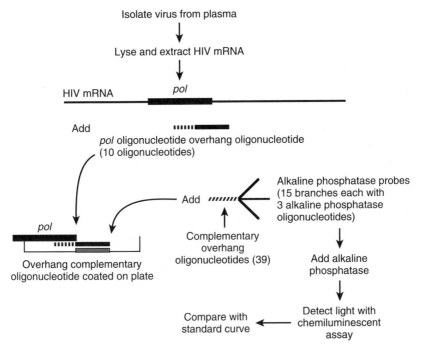

FIGURE 9–5. **The Branched Chain DNA Signal Amplification Assay.** This assay amplifies the alkaline phosphatase readout rather than the HIV mRNA as would be the case with polymerase chain reaction (PCR). The HIV-1 virus is isolated from plasma and HIV-1 RNA is extracted. Oligonucleotides that are complementary to 10 different regions of the *pol* gene of HIV are added to the solution of HIV-1 mRNA. The oligonucleotides hybridize to the pol mRNA. Attached to the pol oligonucleotides is an "overhang" oligonucleotide that is recognized by and binds to a complementary sequence that is coated in microwells on the plate. A second oligonucleotide overhang (39 different oligonucleotides binding to different regions of the first overhang) is added to the reaction. These overhang oligonucleotides have a series of branches with oligonucleotides to alkaline phosphatase. Alkaline phosphatase is added to the mix and a light reaction is generated that is proportional to the amount of pol mRNA that has bound to the first overhang on the plate.

HIV adapted for growth in T-cell lines and HIV obtained from individuals with long-standing, advanced disease could infect T cells and T-cell lines but not macrophages. Thus, there are macrophage-trophic (M-trophic) and T-cell trophic (T-trophic) HIV strains that correspond to early and late strains of HIV. All these findings have suggested the presence of a second receptor on immune cells that interacts with CD4 to provide for cell specificity of HIV cell entry.

Within a several-month period in 1996, a number of articles appeared that identified and characterized two CD4 coreceptors for HIV, identified natural cytokine ligands for these receptors, and defined genetic mutations in one of the receptors that links to resistance to infection from HIV and correlates with prolonged survival once infected. This flurry of activity related to HIV receptors also identified potential new targets for HIV therapy.

The approach to finding the T-trophic CD4 coreceptor used a combination of molecular and cell biology (Fig. 9–6). NIH 3T3 cells, a human fibroblast cell line, were the target cells for this study, whereas HeLa cells, a human epithelial cell, provided the cDNA library that contained the coreceptor gene. One set of 3T3 cells was transfected with the CD4 receptor cDNA; another set of cells was transfected with the HIV env protein that binds to CD4 and its coreceptor. The *env* cDNA cells also contained an *Escherichia coli LacZ* gene so that when the *env* cells bound a CD4-coreceptor complex, the cell turned blue when stained with β-galactosidase. Thus, the presence of blue cells was the assay for cell fusion and the presence of the receptor

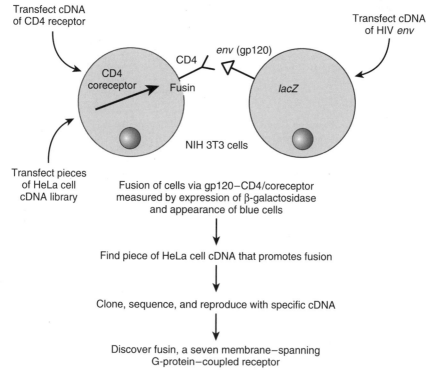

FIGURE 9–6. **Finding Fusin, the T-Trophic CD4 Coreceptor.** NIH 3T3 cells were transfected with either the CD4 receptor or with HIV-1 *env* cDNAs. The *env*-expressing cells also contained the *lacZ* gene. No fusion occurred between the two cells because a CD4 coreceptor was required. The CD4+ cells were then cotransfected with fragments of a HeLa cell cDNA library. Those fragments containing the coreceptor cDNA allowed fusion between the *env*-expressing and CD4-expressing cells. This was measured by a sharp increase in *lacZ*-containing cells, which turned blue in the presence of β-galactoside. The HeLa cell cDNA that increased fusion was cloned and sequenced. The cloned cDNA was retransfected and duplicated the fusion of env and CD4 cells; thus fusin, the T-trophic CD4 coreceptor was discovered.

complex. With this assay in place, the HeLa cell cDNA library, cut into pieces with restriction enzymes, was transfected into the CD4-bearing cells. Transfection of a piece of DNA containing the coreceptor gene was identified when fusion with *env*-expressing cells had increased, as indicated by a blue color in increasing numbers of cells. The piece of cDNA was then cloned and sequenced, and the protein was isolated and studied. The coreceptor proved to be a seven transmembrane–spanning G protein–coupled receptor, which was given the name fusin or CxCR4. It was naturally present in T-trophic, but not in M-trophic, cells; antibodies to the protein blocked HIV fusion and transfection of the fusin, and CD4 cDNAs confirmed fusion potential to a wide variety of cells. The natural ligand for the fusin receptor was not known and it was for some time felt to be an orphan receptor, a receptor without known ligand, although a cytokine SDF1 has recently been identified as the fusin ligand.

Discovery of the second CD4 coreceptor, the M-trophic coreceptor, followed shortly. It had been shown previously that several β-cytokines were capable of suppressing HIV infection of M-cells. These cytokines were known to bind to G protein–coupled receptors similar to fusin. It was also shown that individuals who were resistant to HIV infection tended to have high cirulating levels of β-cytokines. Since the β-cytokine family of receptors had already been described, it was relatively easy to transfect the various cDNAs of known receptors into cells along with CD4 and to determine which receptor conferred HIV env-mediated infectivity to the cells. The coreceptor was found to be CC-CKR-5 (CC is derived from two adjacent cysteines that characterize the receptor and CKR stands for cytokine receptor). Expression of CD4 and CC-CKR-5 in cells allowed the cells to be infected with M-trophic but not T-trophic HIV, and CC-CKR-5 was expressed in monocytes-macrophages and T cells but not T-cell lines.

A fascinating observation was that macrophage-monocytes from exposed but uninfected individuals that could not be infected with M-trophic HIV were rendered infectible by transfection of CC-CKR-5. Exposed but uninfected individuals have had multiple exposures to HIV but are uninfected. It was only a matter of time before the CC-CKR-5 receptor of exposed but uninfected individuals was sequenced and shown to have a mutation that led to a 32–base pair deletion and expression of a truncated protein (CC-CKR-5d32) that had no G protein coupling domain and was not expressed on the cell surface. One percent of the Caucasian population is homozygous for this deletion, and 16 to 20% of this population is heterozygous (i.e., have one abnormal allele). The mutation is not found in black or Japanese populations. A recent study has also shown some correlation between heterozygosity and survival once an individual is infected. The fact that homozygotes for CC-CKR-5d32 have no phenotype and appear to be immunologically normal suggests that HIV infection could be prevented by blocking this receptor without harming the patient.

The picture of HIV infection that derives from these recent observations

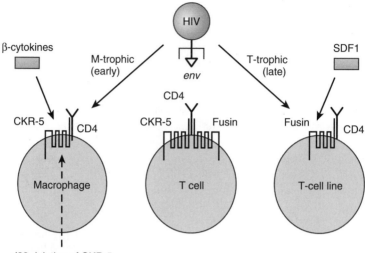

FIGURE 9–7. **HIV-1 Infection of Immune Cells: The Tale of Two Coreceptors.** Early on, HIV-1 env protein (gp120) binds to and infects macrophage-monocytes and T cells via the CD4/ CC-CKR-5 coreceptors. This is the M-trophic virus. As the disease progresses, HIV-1 binds to and infects T cells and T-cell lines via the CD4-fusin coreceptor. Late HIV-1 virus is T-trophic rather than M-trophic. β-Cytokines are the natural ligands for CD4/CC-CKR-5 and block HIV-1 access to the receptor. SDF1 is the natural ligand for the CD4-fusin coreceptor. There appears to be a change in one of the immunoglobulin domains of HIV-1 that is involved in the switch from M- to T-trophic virus. A 32–base pair deletion in the CC-CKR-5 gene results in a truncated nonfunctional coreceptor protein and is associated with resistance to infection with HIV-1 in homozygotes for this deletion and with a more prolonged course of HIV in heterozygotes.

is illustrated in Figure 9–7 (see also Fig. 9–4) Early infection of M cells (macrophage-monocytes and T cells) occurs via CD4 and CC-CKR-5. HIV replicates rapidly, kills CD4 + cells, achieving some plateau level in infected individuals that is determined in part by host responses to the virus and by mutations in the CC-CKR-5 receptor. At some time during the course of infection, the HIV env protein undergoes a change or mutation that allows it now to be T-trophic and infect additional groups of T cells. At this time, the peripheral CD4 count begins to drop, heralding the terminal phase of HIV infection.

## Silicon Chip to DNA Chip: A New Tool for Detecting Drug Resistance and Much More

One of the major concerns in treating AIDS has been the ability of HIV to mutate and become resistant to anti-HIV drugs. The initial wave of anti-HIV drugs were inhibitors of reverse transcriptase. These agents did not actually kiil virus or reverse low CD4+ counts. The hot new drugs are now the antiproteases. HIV produces a protease that is necessary for processing viral proteins into the infectious virus particle. These proteases have been the target of a new line of drugs that inhibit protease activity and viral replication. They have had a huge impact on the treatment of AIDS. However, HIV isolates grown in culture undergo mutations that might foster resistance to antiproteases. Therefore, investigators have begun to survey mutations in protease genes that occur in patients on therapy.

Recently, silicon chip technology has been applied to this problem, and the methods used have also been adapted to screen for mutations in cancer-related genes, to determine the genetic differences between normal and cancer tissue, and for genome sequencing. The method employs silicon chip technology but fixes oligonucleotides instead of electrical circuits to the chips (Fig. 9–8).

One of the first articles published using this technology examined mutations in HIV proteases that appear in HIV-infected individuals who have not yet received antiprotease therapy. Surprisingly, this study showed that the

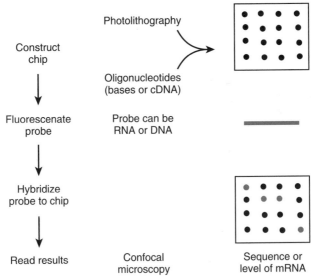

FIGURE 9–8. **DNA Microarray—the "Chip" and HIV.** Silicon chips are etched by photolithography so that oligonucleotides (either single bases or chains) can be attached to the chip. Bases are used for sequencing and searching for gene mutations; oligonucleotides are used to assay changes in gene expression. As many as 100,000 oligonucleotide probes can be placed on a 1.6-cm² chip. The material to be probed by the chip can be RNA or DNA. It is fluorescenated and then hybridized to the chip. During hybridization, interactions between probe and chip occur so that the bases in the probe adhere in a complementary fashion to bases on the chip. The fluorescence on the chip representing intensity of hybridization is read with a scanning confocal microscope, and probe sequence or level of mRNA is calculated.

protease gene *(pr),* even before exposure to antiproteases, was extremely variable, with variations in almost half of the 99 protease amino acids. This finding suggests caution about the use of antiproteases as single therapy, since many amino acid changes known to be associated with drug resistance occur as natural polymorphisms in patients who have never been exposed to antiprotease drugs.

The availability of the DNA chip allowed rapid sequencing on many samples isolated over a short period. For sequencing, each nucleotide in the target (the *pr* gene in this case) is interrogated by a panel of nucleotide probes on the chip. The minimal number of oligonucleotides on the chip is four times the length of the target sequence. Thus each nucleotide in the target sequence is interrogated by an A, T, G, or C on the chip. The material being probed is converted into fluorescein-labeled RNA, and the RNA is fragmented. Following sequence-specific hybridization of the RNA fragments to the chip, the fluorescein-labeled RNA is detected on the surface of the chip using epifluorescence scanning confocal microscopy. The best hybridization—for example, a G to a C—generates the brightest signal. Interrogation of a large number of fragments allows one to determine the full sequence of the RNA being "interrogated." In the case of the *pr* gene, 382 base pairs of HIV, which included the 267–base pair *pr* gene, were subjected to PCR, transcribed into RNA, and sequenced.

As noted earlier, DNA chips have been made with cDNA probes and DNA sequences to detect differences on gene expression in cancer versus noncancer cells. They have also been made with oligonucleotides designed to search for mutations in the *BRCA1* breast cancer gene, and chips for other cancer-related genes are being prepared. Genome sequencing, diagnostics, and genetic mutation detection chips and the accompanying scanning system will likely soon be part of every hospital laboratory.

## SUGGESTED READING

### General

Fauci AS: Host factors and the pathogenesis of HIV-induced disease. Nature 384:529–533, 1996.

### Viral Load

Mellors JW, Rinaldo CR Jr, Gupta P, et al: Prognosis in HIV-1 infection predicted by the quantity of virus in plasma. Science 272:1167–1170, 1996.

Pachl C, Todd JA, Kern DG, et al: Rapid and precise quantification of HIV-1 RNA in plasma using a branched DNA signal amplification assay. J Acquir Immune Defic Syndr Hum Retrovirol 8:446–454, 1995.

Perelson AS, Neumann AU, Markowitz M, et al: HIV-1 dynamics in vivo: Virion clearance rate, infected cell life-span, and viral generation time. Science 271:1582–1586, 1996.

### Human Immunodeficiency Virus as a Gene Delivery Vehicle

Naldini L, Blomer U, Gage FH, et al: In vivo gene delivery and stable transduction of nondividing cells by a lentiviral vector. Science 272:263–267, 1996.

## CD4 Coreceptors

Choe H, Farzan M, Sun Y, et al: The b-cytokine receptors CCR3 and CCR5 facilitate infection by primary HIV-1 isolates. Cell 85:1135–1148, 1996.

Dean M, Carrington M, Winkler C, et al: Genetic restriction of HIV-1 infection and progression to AIDS by a deletion allele of the CKR5 structural gene. Science 273:1856–1862, 1996.

Deng H, Liu R, Ellmeier W, et al: Identification of a major co-receptor for primary isolates of HIV-1. Nature 381:661–666, 1996.

Dragic T, Litwin V, Allway GP, et al: HIV-1 entry into CD4+ cells is mediated by the chemokine receptor CC-CDK-5. Nature 381:667–673, 1996.

Feng Y, Broder CC, Kennedy PE, et al: HIV-1 entry cofactor: Functional cDNA cloning of a seven-transmembrane G protein-coupled receptor. Science 272:872–877, 1996.

Liu R, Paxton WA, Choe S, et al: Homozygous defect in HIV-1 coreceptor accounts for resistance of some multiply-exposed individuals to HIV-1 infection. Cell 86:367–377, 1996.

## DNA Microarray

DeRisi J, Penland L, Brown PO, et al: Use of a cDNA microarray to analyze gene expression patterns in human cancer. Nat Genetics 14:457–460, 1996.

Kozal ML, Shah N, Shen N, et al: Extensive polymorphisms observed in HIV-1 clade B protease gene using high-density oligonucleotide arrays. Nat Med 2:753–759, 1996.

# Back to Genetics: The Human Genome Project and Asthma

sequencing genomes—human and others •
sequence targeted sites and expressed
sequence tags • genetic footprints •
determining gene functions • new life forms
• complex genetic diseases

The Human Genome Project (HGP) was planned in the late 1980s. At the time it seemed like science fiction to most of us. In 1990, specific goals were set forth that were expected to be achieved in part by 2010. The goals were to develop "detailed genetic and physical maps of the human genome, determine the complete nucleotide sequence of human DNA, and develop the new technology necessary to achieve these ambitious goals." To understand how ambitious these goals were, one only has to remember the human genome analogy discussed in Chapter 1; the 3 billion base pairs of the human genome, if assembled as a book, would fill 1000 volumes, each with 1000 pages. The HGP aimed not only to decipher the identity and sequence of the letters on each page and the order of the individual pages but also to include "the construction of detailed genetic and physical maps and acquisition of DNA sequence information characterizing the genomes of several nonhuman organisms. . . ." In 1995 to 1996, the publication of the first almost-complete genetic physical map and completion of DNA sequencing of several bacteria and one yeast organism and a worm genome were accomplished. The progress has been amazing, and as a result the goals of the HGP are continually being redefined and upgraded, and the date for complete sequencing has been moved forward by at least 5 years.

As with the story of cystic fibrosis and positional cloning, the rapid progress on the HGP required new technical advances and new ideas and the emergence of new informatics technology to deal with the overwhelming amount of data being generated. Two very different approaches have been used, based on different principles but providing complementary results (Fig. 10–1). Recently, a map was published that covers 95% of the whole genome. This map includes sequence information of 200 to 500 base pairs, each spread over 15,000 sites on the 23 human chromosomes, at average intervals 200 kb apart. The initial goal for physical maps was 30,000 sites at intervals of 100 kb, so the map is more than half finished. It took 15 million polymerase chain reactions (PCR) and a team of 25 individuals 2.5 years to get this far. In addition, information from work by a number of investigators was used.

Figure 10–2 outlines the general methods used to establish the present physical genetic map. The approach involved a human genomic library, establishing PCR primers from a variety of sources, and mapping sequence targeted sites using concepts related to genetic recombination and linkage analysis, which were covered in Chapter 3. It should take another year or so to double

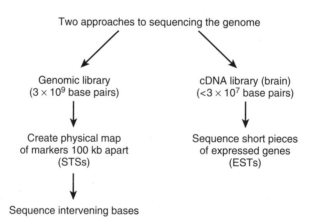

FIGURE 10–1. **The Two Major Approaches to Sequencing the Human Genome.** The Human Genome Project (HGP) approach *(left side of figure)* provides a physical map of the genome followed in time with a complete reading of genomic DNA. The expressed sequence tag *(ESTs)* approach *(right side of figure)* involves random sequencing of pieces of cDNA and is thus tissue-specific and time-specific and depends on where and when various mRNAs are expressed. STSs, sequence targeted sites.

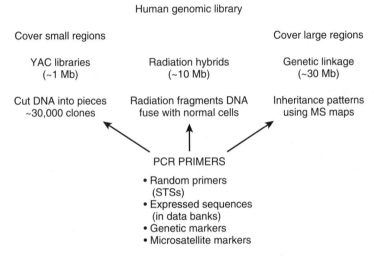

Human genomic library

Cover small regions                                      Cover large regions

YAC libraries          Radiation hybrids          Genetic linkage
(~1 Mb)                    (~10 Mb)                   (~30 Mb)

Cut DNA into pieces   Radiation fragments DNA   Inheritance patterns
~30,000 clones         fuse with normal cells        using MS maps

PCR PRIMERS

- Random primers
  (STSs)
- Expressed sequences
  (in data banks)
- Genetic markers
- Microsatellite markers

Analyze which PCR products segregate with one another

Build independent maps

Combine to produce integrated map

FIGURE 10–2. **The Human Genome Project: Generating a Physical-Genetic Map.** Following construction of a human genomic DNA library, restriction enzymes are used to cut DNA into pieces that are packaged in yeast artificial chromosomes *(YAC)* that can hold 1 Mb of contiguous DNA. A second approach has been to put pieces of DNA into cells that are then subjected to radiation, which fragments the DNA. The fragmented DNA is saved by fusion with normal cells, with the DNA closest together in the genome tending to appear in the same cell. PCR primers from a number of different sources (including random primers that identify sequence tagged sites *[STSs]*) are used to determine which sequences appear linked, that is, in the same cells or associated with the same markers. Physical maps from each system are constructed, and then the three maps are combined to produce the final product. This process involved more than 15 million polymerase chain reaction *(PCR)* effects and required extensive informatics technology. The map and primer sites are available on the Internet. MS, microsatellite.

the number of sites and to shorten the distance between them to the target 100-kb distance. This map provides the scaffold for the difficult technical task remaining—that of sequencing everything in between the sequence targeted sites. After this has been accomplished—that is, all the human genes have been discovered—the big problem of determining gene function remains.

Another approach to human genome sequencing has been to reason that since more than 95% of the genome is not transcribed into mRNA, why not concentrate on the translated products and ignore the "junk DNA"? This would mean that only cDNAs would be sequenced. This approach requires extraction of mRNA from a tissue and construction of a cDNA library using reverse-transcribed-PCR. Random PCR priming reactions are then used to generate pieces of DNA that can then be sequenced. These products are called expressed sequence tags and they can ultimately be used to clone, fully sequence, and locate tissue-specific genes. This approach is much faster in that much of the genome is ignored; only small pieces of cDNA need be sequenced, and ordered location of the cDNA pieces is not required. However, much time and tissue-specific information is not obtained by this approach, and genes of low abundance tend to be missed. As of mid-1995, 5 million bases of cDNA had been sequenced. This represents less than 0.2% of the genome. However, this small amount of sequenced DNA includes pieces of 50,000 genes, only 20% of which had previously been described. The power of this method is to find pieces of new genes; it does not create a map of the genome.

Computer technology has been crucial in generating genome maps and in creating robotics for the multiple PCR effects involved. One of the additional great benefits of the computer age is that all of this information is now available to all investigators at various Internet locations. In addition, many programs are available that help one search data bases and analyze gene structure and function. What remains is an enormous amount of work to fill in the spaces on the genome map and the even greater task of determining function of the many genes whose function is not predictable with our present state of knowledge.

## Sequencing Other Genomes: Rapid Progress, Many Surprises

The sequencing of other genomes is also ahead of schedule. Several bacteria have been fully sequenced (*Haemophilus influenzae* and *Mycoplasma genitalium*), as has one yeast (*Saccharomyces cerevisiae*), and the worm *Caenorhabditis elegans.* Work on several other genomes is in progress, and a physical map of the mouse genome has been produced.

What has been learned from these studies? Figure 10–3 demonstrates one consistent finding: the simpler the organism, the smaller the genome and the more dense the organization of genes on chromosomes. Said another way,

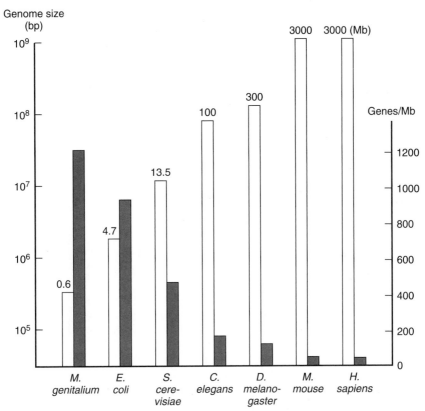

FIGURE 10–3. **Species Comparison of Genome Size and Density: Evolution Adds Junk.** Graph of genome size *(open bars)* versus density of genes on chromosomes *(gray-shaded),* for seven different species *(Mycoplasma genitalium, Escherichia coli, Saccharomyces cerevisiae, Caenorhabditis elegans, Drosophila melanogaster, Mus musculis mouse,* and *Homo sapiens).* Mice and humans have the lowest density of genes per length of genomic DNA and thus have more regulatory, intronic, and repeat sequences than do lower species. The function of all this extra DNA remains uncertain. bp, base pair.

simple organisms have less junk. As a result, genes are packed into a smaller space; 97% of the human genome is thought to represent junk, that is, intronic and upstream regulatory information, microsatellite repeats, and so on. The observation that the higher the organism the more the junk points to accumulation of junk as an important clue to evolution. It is obvious that gene duplication and redundancy of gene function are associated with evolution; human genes often have multiple overlapping functions.

The smallest genome that has been fully sequenced is that of *M. genitalium.* It has only 482 genes, with 30% of them having sequences consistent with being integral membrane proteins and thus being dedicated to regulating the interaction of this bacterium with its environment. It is rather disconcerting to find that there is no clue as to the function of more than 20% of the genes in this simple organism. A similar picture evolves from sequencing the S. *cerevisiae* genome. Despite extensive use of this organism in biologic research, the function of 40% of its 6000 genes remains a mystery; there is no clue from sequence homologies as to their functions. The good news in the comparisons of the genome of lower organisms and humans is the conservation of gene function. Many homologs of human genes have been found in yeast and bacteria, thus providing simple experimental organisms to explore gene function.

## All Those Genes and No Function: Genetic Footprinting

As noted, all the genome sequencing has resulted in a lot of genes with no known function. Some functions can be implied through sequence homologies with genes in other species. However, determining gene function remains a major challenge for gene sequencers.

A clever new approach to determining gene function in yeast may prove applicable to the increasing list of mammalian genes that have been discovered but have no known function. The method, called genome footprinting, involves insertional mutagenesis, growth selection, and PCR analysis of gene disruption (Fig. 10–4). In these experiments, a marked transposon element, Ty1 (see Chapter 2), was randomly induced to undergo transposition in yeast, inserting at many places in the genome and thereby, in many but not all cases, interrupting expression of genes and their functions. Yeasts were then subjected to a variety of growth media, and their ability to proliferate under different growth conditions was evaluated. DNA from yeast that responded differently to the growth conditions was isolated and subjected to PCR with primers for Ty1 and for sequences of recently described genes on yeast chromosome V. The PCR footprint before and after Ty1 transpositions allowed identification of where the Ty1-induced deletions were located, and these gene deletions could then be correlated with altered cell "fitness." Specific gene mutations could be assigned to mutant phenotypes, and conditions to explore exact gene functions could be defined. This approach has a good chance of defining functions for the 40% of yeast genes without any known species sequence homologies. Once functions are assigned, similar genes in other species can be sought.

## A New Life Form from the Depths

The biggest surprise in species genome sequencing came in the summer of 1996 when the complete genome of *Methanococcus jannaschii* was published. Its genome has provided firm evidence of a life form that lies between

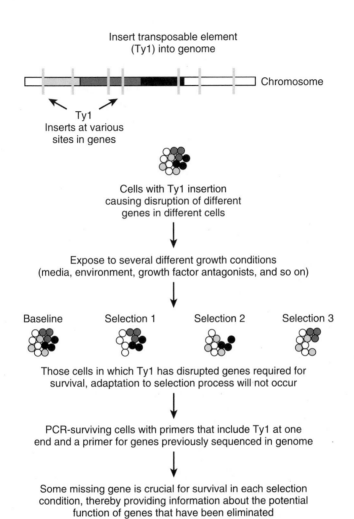

FIGURE 10–4. **Determining Gene Function by Genetic Footprinting.** The transposon Ty1 can be induced to insert at many sites in the yeast genome. In some instances, these elements disrupt gene translation or function. In this method, cells with various genes disrupted are exposed to different growth conditions. Those yeasts with dysfunctional genes that are required for adaptation to the altered conditions will die. If one performs PCR with the DNA of surviving cells with a Ty1 primer and with a primer that is gene-specific, the gene or genes that have been disrupted and are crucial for survival will no longer be present and the DNA footprint of the cells will be altered; some DNA will be missing. The function of that gene in assisting survival can then be explored in detail.

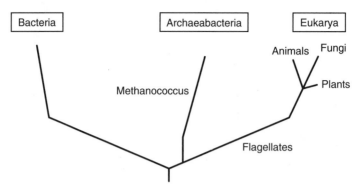

FIGURE 10–5. **A New Life Form Domain from the Ocean Depths.** Sequencing the genome of *Methanococcus jannaschii* found in hydrothermal areas at ocean depths has firmly established a domain that lies between prokaryotic bacteria and eukaryotes, which include humans. The Archaeabacteria genome contains genes homologous to those in both prokaryotes and eukaryotes as well as a large number of genes unlike any that have been described to date.

prokaryotes (bacteria that do not contain a nucleus) and eukaryotes (organisms with a nucleus, including animals). rRNA sequencing differences had already established that there might be three life form domains: the prokaryotes, a form of bacteria called Archaeabacteria that live at extremes of temperature and pressure and that metabolize sulfur and hydrogen, and eukaryotes (Fig. 10–5). *M. jannaschii* was found 3 km below the ocean surface around the opening to hydrothermal chimneys on the ocean floor. Sequencing the genome of these recently discovered methane-producing organisms established that they had similarities to both prokaryotes and eukaryotes. As an example, they contained a number of histone genes similar to those in animals. The histones are involved in the tight packaging of DNA on chromosomes. This organism also contained genes involved in energy metabolism, transcription, translation, and replication similar to eukaryotes, yet contained genes related to energy production, cell division, and metabolism that resembled the prokaryotes. Of great interest was the fact that more than 60% of the organism's 1738 putative genes were unrelated to anything ever sequenced before. Thus genome sequencing has confirmed the presence of a new life form domain and has presented investigators with a large number of genes whose functions remain to be determined and may provide new information about evolution.

## Asthma: An Example of a Complex Genetic Disease

Asthma is a disease that in most instances has genetic roots. Numerous studies, in twins and in families, have documented that it is a heritable disease. However, it differs from diseases caused by a single dominant, recessive, or sex-linked gene defect, such as sickle cell anemia, cystic fibrosis, amyotrophic lateral sclerosis, and hemophilia. Asthma fits into the category of complex genetic diseases such as hypertension, atherosclerosis, and diabetes in which heredity clearly plays a role but inheritance does not follow a simple mendelian pattern.

Complex genetic diseases tend to be more prevalent in the general population than do simple mendelian diseases. For example, asthma occurs in 4 to 8% of the general population, whereas cystic fibrosis occurs in 0.05% of the white population. Complex genetic diseases are complex because defects in different genes may result in disease, because different combinations of gene defects may result in disease, or because gene defects and the environment may interact to produce disease. It seems likely that all these conditions occur in asthma.

Although it has been known for years that there is a heritable basis to asthma, it has been a particularly difficult disease to study because of its variable phenotype. By comparison, hypertension has a simple phenotype: elevated blood pressure, although even in this case diastolic versus systolic and intermittent versus sustained blood pressure elevations confound genetic studies. With asthma, the phenotype is wheezing. However, all that wheezes is not asthma and all asthma does not wheeze. The more precise definition of asthma is reversible airway obstruction together with airway hyperreactivity, a definition that is much more difficult to measure than is hypertension. Even this definition has limitations because other diseases that cause airway inflammation (such as viral infections) result in hyperreactivity. It is generally felt that asthma has an allergic component, yet how this is assessed (skin tests, IgE levels, history) will affect the phenotype. In addition, asthma can be present without allergic manifestations. It seems reasonable to postulate that the asthma phenotype that is investigated might influence the gene identified. Certainly the variability of the phenotype suggests that multiple interacting factors are involved and that asthma is indeed a complex genetic disease.

To date, most genetic studies of asthma have focused on "allergic" asthma. The molecular techniques used in these studies tend to be similar to the linkage analysis studies discussed in Chapter 3: phenotypic markers are linked to genotypic markers by analysis of large cohorts. Different approaches to finding the asthma gene and the genetic methods used are discussed in detail in two recent reviews and an excellent review of the basic science of complex genetic diseases. In general, what differs in various studies is the population being studied and the focus of the gene search. The most ambitious studies now under way survey whole populations that are being extensively characterized, with the focus on a broad-based search of the whole genome for linkage. In this instance, genome screening uses the multiple microsatellite markers that have been described with automated robotic PCR and DNA analysis. Other studies involve specific well-defined populations, such as sibs with asthma or asthmatic individuals with elevated IgE levels.

TABLE 10–1
***Examples of Putative Asthma Gene Locations***

| Site | Phenotype | Putative Gene |
| --- | --- | --- |
| 5q31 | IgE level | Cytokine gene cluster (IL4, |
|  | Airway hyperreactivity | IL5, IL13, GM-CSF) |
| 5q32-34 | Asthma severity (nocturnal asthma) | $\beta_2$-Adrenergic receptor |
| 6 | Allergens and HLA haplotype |  |
| 11q13 | Maternal inheritance | High-affinity IgE receptor |
| 14q | IgE responses | T-cell receptor |

A specific mutation in the IL4 promoter has been identified that results in increased IL4 transcription. A substitution of a glycine at position 16 for an arginine results in accelerated agonist down-regulation of the beta receptor associated with nocturnal asthmatics.

IL4, interleukin 4; GM-CSF, granulocyte macrophage–colony stimulating factor.

Gene searches have been broad-based or focused, for example, to loci known to code for inflammatory cytokines. Some searches have focused on mutations in specific genes thought to be involved in asthma, for example, the $\beta_2$-adrenergic receptor. Some of the results of these studies are summarized in Table 10–1.

Many studies are now in progress. They will likely focus further on defects in specific known genes or, in the case of genome searches, discover new genes that may play crucial roles in asthma. Given the complex genetic nature of the disease, it is unlikely that a single "asthma gene" will be found that defines *the* cause of asthma. What all investigators hope is that genes that are causally linked to asthma will provide insights into its pathophysiology and provide clues for the design of new agents for treating or preventing asthma.

## SUGGESTED READING

### Human Genome Project

Collins FS: Ahead of schedule and under budget: The genome project passes its fifth birthday. Proc Natl Acad Sci 92:10821–10823, 1995. [associated review articles]

Hudson TJ, Stein LD, Gerety SS, et al: An STS-based map of the human genome. Science 270:1945–1954, 1995. [accompanying editorial]

### Genomes of Other Species

Bult CJ, White O, Olsen GJ, et al: Complete genome sequence of the methanogenic archaeon, *Methanococcus jannaschii.* Science 273:1058–1073, 1996. [accompanying editorial]

Goffeau A: Life with 482 genes. Science 270:445–446, 1995. [several accompanying articles on species genome sequencing]

Smith V, Chou KN, Lashkari D, et al: Functional analysis of the genes of yeast chromosome V by genetic footprinting. Science 274:2069–2074, 1996.

## Asthma: A Complex Genetic Disease

Bleecker ER, Meyers DA: Genetics of allergy and asthma. *In* Kay BA (ed): Allergy. Oxford, England, Blackwell Scientific, 1996, pp 1194–1205.

Lander ES, Schrock NJ: Genetic dissection of complex traits. Science 265:2037–2048, 1994. [accompanying editorial comment]

Sandford A, Weir T, Pare P: The genetics of asthma. Am J Respir Crit Care Med 153:1749–1765, 1996.

Turki J, Green SA, Martin RJ, et al: Genetic polymorphisms of the beta 2-adrenergic receptor in nocturnal and non-nocturnal asthma. Evidence that Gly 16 correlates with nocturnal phenotype. J Clin Invest 95:1635–1641, 1995.

# Glossary

. . . . . . . . . . . . . . . . . . . . .

**Acceptor site:** An AG sequence defining the splice site at the 3′ end of an intron.

**Allele:** The different forms that a segment of DNA or a gene has in a population; in an individual, one allele of a gene is inherited from each parent.

**Alternative splicing:** Primary gene transcripts that can be spliced in different ways to create two different mRNAs and, on occasion, two different proteins.

**Amino acid:** The fundamental building blocks of a protein, which are encoded by one or more triplet codons. There are a total of 20 amino acids.

**Amino terminus (N terminus):** The end of a polypeptide chain that carries a free amino group.

**Anaphase:** A stage of cell division in which sister chromatids separate and move to opposite ends of the nucleus.

**Anticodons:** Complementary nucleotide sequences in tRNA that allow its binding to specific sequences of mRNA.

**Antisense RNA:** RNA that is complementary to mRNA that can specifically bind to and block function of that RNA.

**Antisense (strands):** The noncoding strands of DNA complementary to the sense (coding) strands. The antisense strand is the strand that produces mRNA.

**Apoptosis:** A regulated process of programmed cell death.

**Bacteriophage:** A virus that can infect and multiply in bacteria. Foreign DNA can be inserted into phage, which can then be grown in bacteria.

**Base pair (bp):** Complimentary bases in double-stranded DNA; A-T, G-C.

**Blunt ends:** The two chains of DNA cut by restriction enzymes that leave no overhang, that is, ends are evenly cut.

**Candidate gene:** A gene thought to be responsible for a disease or a biologic phenomenon on the basis of its properties or its protein product.

**Capsid:** The external protein coat of a viral particle, usually in the form of a geometric structure.

**Cassette:** A DNA fragment that carries the desired sequences to be inserted into a vector for subsequent transfection.

**cDNA library:** A set of cloned fragments of DNA that has been derived by reverse-transcribing mRNA into DNA.

**Cell lines (immortalized cells):** Cells that grow indefinitely in culture. Many cell lines are derived from tumors or have cell cycle regulatory genes that have been inactivated.

**Centromere:** The region of the chromosome that separates its two arms.

**CG island:** Unmethylated CG nucleotides often found near the 5′ ends of many genes.

**Chromatin:** The combination of proteins and DNA that make up chromosomes.

**Chromosome:** A structure that carries the species' genes; it is made up of long pieces of double-stranded DNA and proteins. Chromosomes are visible during cell division when they segregate and become condensed in the nucleus.

**Chromosome walking:** The process by which one sequences overlapping chromosomal clones progressing toward a gene of interest.

***cis*-Acting factors or elements:** The specific DNA base sequences in a gene that serve as binding sites for transcription factors that regulate transcription of DNA into RNA.

**Clone:** A large number of cells or molecules such as DNA that are identical and stem from a common precursor.

**Cloning:** A means of isolating clones of cells or molecules, usually growing large numbers of cells (often expressing a specific molecule of piece of DNA) from a single precursor.

**Codon:** A sequence of three nucleotides in mRNA that provides information that is necessary for incorporation of a specific amino acid in the peptide chain assembling on the ribosome as a protein is produced.

**Complementary:** The pairing of bases, dictated by spatial and energetic factors that result from hydrogen bonds, resulting in preferential pairing of A with T or U (in RNA) and C with G in DNA.

**Complementary DNA or cDNA:** DNA molecule that is made as a copy of mRNA. It does not contain the 5′ flanking regions and intronic sequences of genomic DNA.

**Consensus sequence:** The idealized or most typical sequence depicting the nucleotide or amino acid most often appearing in DNA or a protein molecule.

**Contigs:** Contiguous stretches of DNA assembled in correct order from DNA fragments within a single vector.

**Cosmids:** Hybrid vectors into which one can insert approximately 45 kb of DNA.

**Cotransfection:** Simultaneous transfection of two different DNA species into a cell.

**Crossing over:** The exchange of genetic material between homologous chromosomes that occurs during meiosis and occasionally during mitosis. It is this process that is responsible for homologous recombination and is the basis of gene knockout technology.

**Degenerate:** Refers to the fact that several triplet nucleotide sequences can code for the same amino acid (see Fig. 1–8). Thus, constructing a degenerate oligonucleotide to probe for an amino acid sequence requires one to take this redundancy into account.

**Deletion:** Removal of a portion of DNA with the regions on either side being joined together.

**Denature:** To change the structure of a molecule, most often by subjecting it to heat or chemicals.

**Diploid:** Human cells have two copies of each chromosome; the diploid number is 46. Sex cells (gametes) have a haploid number of chromosomes (23).

**Divergent:** Expressing the difference in nucleotide or amino acid sequence between two DNAs or two proteins.

**DNA:** The double helical molecule consisting of a sugar backbone and four bases that codes for mRNA.

**DNA fingerprint:** Pieces of DNA that have been cut by restriction enzymes, separated on a gel, and identified with a labeled complementary probe. If the probe is highly polymorphic, the resulting pattern of DNA (fingerprint) will be specific for an individual or an organism.

**DNA polymerase:** An enzyme involved in DNA replication.

**DNA repair:** A process by which errors made in replication of DNA during the cell cycle are altered so as to preserve the fidelity of new DNA.

**Dominant:** An allele that is expressed in the same fashion whether it is in a heterozygous or homozygous form. The opposite of recessive.

**Dominant negative:** An altered protein (either arising spontaneously or produced intentionally) that acts to suppress the function of the normal protein.

**Donor site:** The sequence GT that defines the splice site at the 5′ end of an intron.

**Dot blots:** mRNA not separated by electrophoresis is placed on a filter for subsequent hybridization with a labeled oligonucleotide probe.

**Electrophoresis:** A technique in which charged molecules are placed in a medium and are separated in an electrical field primarily on the basis of size.

**Embryonic stem cell:** Cell derived from a blastocyst, having the capacity to differentiate into any lineage. These cells are used primarily for production of null mutant mice.

**Endonucleases:** Enzymes that cleave bonds within a nucleic acid chain.

**Enhancer:** A protein that binds to a specific DNA site, increasing the level of transcription of a gene. Enhancers are capable of increasing gene expression whether they are upstream or downstream of the promoter and in any orientation.

**Eukaryote:** An organism whose cells have true nuclei.

**Exon:** Portions of genes that are retained in processed mRNA.

**Exonucleases:** Enzymes that cleave nucleotides at the end of a chain.

**Expression library:** A set of cloned fragments of cDNA that effectively translate mRNA into secreted proteins.

**Expression vector:** A vector that contains elements, such as a poly A tail to stabilize mRNA, to support expression of cloned cDNA.

**5′ and 3′:** Carbon atoms in each sugar (ribose for RNA and deoxyribose for DNA) are numbered beginning at the end closest to the aldehyde or ketone. The 1′ carbon of nucleic acids links to a base, the 3′ carbon connects to the phosphate group attached to the 5′ carbon of the preceding nucleic acid, and so on (see Fig. 1–3). The 3′ end of a series or chain of nucleic acids has a hydroxyl group, and the 5′ end has a phosphate group. This numbering system provides a road map for DNA and RNA; for example, the promoter of a gene lies 5′ to the transcription start site and DNA is transcribed by RNA polymerase in a 5′ to 3′ direction.

**5′ Cap site:** A modified guanine nucleotide that is added to and stabilizes the 5′ end of an mRNA being transcribed.

**5′ Flanking region:** That portion of genomic DNA that lies upstream—that is, 5′—from the transcription initiation site. The 5′ flanking region contains regulatory elements, including the promoter, which determine under what circumstances DNA is transcribed.

**FISH or fluorescence in situ hybridization:** A cytogenetic method for visualizing the site at which a gene is present on a chromosome. It involves hybridizing a labeled probe with a chromosomal preparation that is then visualized by fluorescence microscopy.

**Footprint:** Visualization of proteins bound to DNA by virtue of proteins protecting DNA from degradation by endonucleases.

**Fusion gene or protein:** A combination of two or more genes or parts of genes that produces a new protein.

**Gene:** A segment of DNA sufficient to provide the information for making a specific protein. This includes all the contiguous DNA within that region, including coding as well as regulatory information. It is estimated that there are between 50,000 and 100,000 human genes.

**Gene family:** A group of genes that share similar exon sequences and evolve from the same parent gene. Functions of gene family members are similar, for example, transcription factors, growth factors, and so on.

**Gene therapy:** Insertion of a gene into a cell to correct or treat a hereditary or acquired abnormality. The gene can be directed to a germ cell, thereby correcting the defect in all cells, or to a somatic cell, correcting the defect only in that cell or its progeny.

**Genetic code:** The combination of three nucleotides that signifies an amino acid.

**Genetic engineering:** Altering the genetic makeup of a cell or organism using recombinant DNA technology.

**Genetic marker:** A polymorphic probe, such as a microsatellite repeat or an RFLP, that is linked to a disease locus.

**Genome:** The total of all the DNA of an organism.

**Genomic DNA:** All the DNA, including intronic DNA and DNA that regulates gene expression. Not all genomic DNA is transcribed into mRNA.

**Genomic library:** A set of cloned fragments of DNA that represent the entire genome of an organism.

**Genotype:** The genetic makeup of an individual, described by an individual's allelles at a chromosomal site.

**Germ line:** Cells that are responsible for production of one's sex cells (gametes).

**Haploid:** Cells having one copy of chromosomes.

**Heterogeneous RNA or hnRNA:** The nuclear RNA that is an exact copy of DNA; it is processed by removing DNA regulatory sequences and introns to form mRNA, which is then transported to the cytoplasm.

**Heterozygous:** Having two different alleles at a given locus, versus homozygous.

**Homeobox:** The conserved sequence of genes that are homologous to pattern-related transcription factors found in *Drosophila*.

**Homeotic genes:** Genes which, when misexpressed, have the potential of converting one body part into another.

**Homologous:** DNA, chromosomes, or amino acids that are similar to one another.

**Homologous recombination:** Recombination occurs primarily in meiotic cell divisions when pieces of DNA cross over and exchange between chromosomes. When the crossover occurs between similar sites on the chromosome (a relatively rare event), it is called homologous recombination.

**Homozygous:** Having two identical alleles at a given locus.

**Hotspot:** A chromosomal site at which the frequency of DNA mutations is much greater than normal.

**Housekeeping gene:** A gene that is consitutively expressed in all cells because it provides for a basic function carried out in all cells.

**Hybridization:** The formation of hydrogen bonds between complimentary bases A-T and C-G, creating a stable interaction between DNA chains or between DNA or RNA and, for example, a series of manufactured oligonucleotides that are labeled as in Southern or Northern blots.

**Hydropathy plot:** The sequential hydrophobicity of a protein representing the likelihood of its being within a membrane.

**Hydrophilic:** Chemical groups that interact with water to exist within an aqueous environment.

**Hydrophobic:** Chemical groups that repel water and exist within a nonaqueous environment.


**Imprinting:** A change in a gene that results from maternal or paternal alleles expressing vastly different properties, usually as a result of differences in DNA methylation.

**Inducer:** A small molecule, usually a protein, that turns on expression of a gene by binding to either DNA or an associated protein.

**Initiation factors:** Proteins that associate with the ribosome at the beginning of protein synthesis.

**In situ hybridization:** Binding of labeled oligonucleotide to mRNA on a section of tissue or a pellet of cells. Recognition of an mRNA at its site of expression via a hybridization reaction.

**Integration:** Insertion of viral or another DNA sequence into the host genome.

**Interphase:** The period between various stages such as $G_1$, S, and M during cell proliferation.

**Intron:** The DNA between two exons, ultimately spliced out in the processing to mature mRNA.


**Kilobase (kb):** An abbreviation signifying 1000 base pairs of DNA or RNA.

**Knockout:** A null mutation in DNA that eliminates expression of a specific gene.

**Lagging strand:** The alternate strand of DNA that is synthesized during DNA replication.

**λ phage:** A vector capable of containing approximately 15 kb of DNA.

**Lariat:** An intermediate in RNA splicing in which a circular structure is created that leads to elimination of RNA during splicing.

**Linkage:** The tendency of genes to be inherited together as a result of their being close together on the same chromosome; this is true when recombination frequency is less than 50%.

**Linkage disequilibrium:** Nonrandom association of alleles based on their chromosomal proximity, implying that the markers are coordinately inherited.

**Linkage map:** A chart that locates genes and associated markers on the 23 pairs of chromosomes.

**Linker:** A sequence added to a piece of DNA, making it easier to work with. Examples include new restriction sites and make blunt of staggered ended DNA fragments.

**Locus:** The chromosomal location of a specific gene.

**LOD score:** A measure of genetic linkage; the logarithm of the ratio of the likelihood of linkage of a specific recombination fraction to the likelihood of no linkage. A LOD score of 3 is the conventional threshold for linkage.

**Long terminal repeat (LTR):** A sequence repeated at both ends of viral DNA that is a strong transcriptional promoter.

**Loss of heterozygocity (LOH):** A locus at which a deletion or other process has converted a polymorphic (heterozygous) site to one that expresses only a single allele (i.e., is hemizygous).

**Marker:** Polymorphic alleles such as microsatellites that are linked to a disease locus.

**Megabase:** One million base pairs.

**Meiosis:** Cell division in which haploid gametes with 23 chromosomes are formed from diploid cells that contain 46 chromosomes.

**Mendelian:** Describes inheritance of a trait that can be attributed to a single gene.

**Metaphase:** A stage of cell division in which homologous chromosomes are arranged opposite one another in the center of the cell.

**Methylation:** Addition of methyl groups to cytosine groups in GC-rich regions of DNA; correlates with reduced transcription of genes.

**Microsatellite:** Small repeat units of DNA (di-, tri-, tetranucleotides) that occur in tandem throughout the genome. The microsatellites are inherited and can be used as polymorphic genetic markers.

**Mismatch:** The presence of a base in one strand of DNA that is not complementary to the corresponding base of the other strand.

**Mitosis:** The cell division process by which two identical cells are produced from a single parent.

**Mobile elements (transposons):** DNA sequences that can insert themselves into various regions of the genome.

**Mosaic:** The existence of two or more genetically different cells in the same individual.

**Motif:** Short, highly conserved sequences of DNA or RNA, consensus sequences, that represent common functions in different genes, for example, a transcription factor binding site motif. Motifs are used for the construction of databases that extrapolate about DNA or protein functions.

**mRNA or messenger RNA:** The RNA that carries the genetic code directing synthesis of a protein on ribosomes in the cytoplasm. It is a direct copy of DNA, but with introns and regulatory regions of DNA removed.

**Multifactorial:** Traits or diseases that result from the interaction of several genetic or environmental factors.

**Mutations:**

> **Frameshift mutation:** An insertion or deletion of bases that is not a multiple of three, resulting in a change in the sequence of bases and production of a different protein.

> **Insertion-deletion mutation:** A mutation in one or more base pairs that alters the amino acid sequence of a protein.

> **Missense mutations:** Result in a change of an amino acid.

> **Nonsense mutations:** Result in the appearance of a stop codon that prematurely ends translation of an mRNA.

> **Point mutations:** The change in a single nucleotide, which may result in no alteration in amino acid sequence or in a missense or nonsense mutation.

**Northern blot:** mRNA fragments separated by electrophoresis in a gel and transferred (blotted) to some sort of filter for subsequent hybridization with a labeled oligonucleotide probe.

**Nucleotide repeats:** Sequences of nucleotides that appear over and over again (in tandem) throughout the genome. They are usually runs of di-, tri-, or more nucleotides that appear in introns and serve as genomic markers. They have proved to be of value in RFLPs, measures of loss of heterozygocity, and linkage analysis because these repeats are inherited.

**Nucleotides:** 5-Carbon sugar (ribose or deoxyribose), phosphate, and purine or pyrimidine base that are the building blocks of nucleic acid chains. The sugar in DNA is deoxyribose, that in RNA is ribose. The bases in DNA are adenine (A), guanine (G), cytosine (C), and thymidine (T); RNA contains uracil (U) instead of thymidine.

**Null mutation:** See knockout—a mutation that leads to the complete elimination of a gene.

**Oligonucleotide:** A short DNA sequence of nucleotide bases.

**Oncogene:** A gene whose products can transform a cell so that they can grow in an autologous fashion.

**Open reading frame:** The coding sequence of mRNA; that portion of mRNA that encodes the actual protein. It begins with an ATG (methionine, start codon) sequence and ends with a stop codon sequence, UAA,UAG,UGA, that does not code for an amino acid.

**Origin of replication:** The site at which synthesis of DNA begins during its replication.

**Palindrome:** A sequence of DNA that is the same when one strand is read 5' to 3' and the other is read 3' to 5'.

**Penetrance:** The proportion of a population having a disease-causing gene that actually express the disease. If the defective gene is present, but the disease is not expressed, the genotype is of variable or low penetrance.

**Phenotype:** The observed characteristics of an organism or individual, resulting from its genetic makeup.

**Physical map:** Distances between genes or markers on chromosomes.

**Plasmid:** A small circular DNA molecule that can replicate on its own; plasmids are used as vectors for transfer of DNA into cells.

**Poly A tail:** Most mRNAs have a run of adenines at their 3' end, creating a poly A tail. The function of the poly A tail is not known.

**Polygenic:** A disease or trait caused by the combined effect of several genes.

**Polylinker:** A site in a vector that contains many restriction enzyme sequences that appear only once in that vector. The polylinker alllows one to ligate DNA using a variety of enzymes.

**Polymerase chain reaction (PCR):** A method that allows one to amplify many copies of selected DNA targets by repeated cycles of denaturation, annealing of a primer, and extension using a heat-resistant DNA polymerase.

**Polymorphic:** A locus with two or more alleles in a large percentage of the population.

**Polypeptide:** Amino acids linked together by peptide bonds most often forming a protein.

**Polyploidy:** Having more than the normal set of 23 chromosomes in a cell.

**Positional cloning:** The identification and cloning of a gene by determining its physical location.

**Post-translational modification:** Additions or alterations of a polypeptide (e.g., glycosylation, phosphorylation, cleavage) after translation of the mRNA has been completed.

**Primer:** An oligonucleotide that is paired with one strand of DNA, providing a site for DNA polymerase to begin DNA synthesis, as in PCR.

**Probe:** Usually a piece of DNA, RNA, or an oligonucleotide that hybridizes to a target and has a radioactive or colorimetric readout that allows quantitation.

**Promoters:** Nucleotide sequence of DNA to which RNA polymerase binds in order to begin transcription of DNA into RNA; it is within a few bases of the transcription start site.

**Proto-oncogene:** A gene whose protein product is involved in the stimulation of normal cell growth.

**Pseudogene:** A gene that is similar to an active gene but has undergone mutations that have made it inactive.

**Pulse field electrophoresis:** A type of electrophoresis that allows movement of large DNA fragments in a gel.

**Purine:** Bases in DNA and RNA (adenine and guanine) that consist of double carbon-nitrogen rings.

**Pyrimidine:** Bases in DNA (cytosine and thymidine) or RNA (cytosine and uracil) that consist of a single carbon-nitrogen ring.


**Reading frame:** The sequential triplet nucleotides that are the codons for amino acids. A shift in one nucleotide alters the reading frame.

**Recessive:** An allele that is expressed only in the homozygous state.

**Recombination:** The occurrence of new combinations of alleles that occurs as a result of crossing over during meiosis.

**Repetitive DNA:** DNA sequences that are found as multiple copies within the genome.

**Replication fork:** The point at which the two strands of DNA separate so that replication can proceed.

**Reporter gene:** A readout system incorporated into a transfected piece of DNA that provides a signal when the DNA has been transcribed. Commonly used reporter genes include *LacZ,* which produces a blue color in the presence of β-galactoside; luciferase, which produces light in the presence of adenosine triphosphate; and *CAT,* an enzyme, chloramphenicol acetyltransferase, that metabolizes a radiolabeled chloramphenicol substrate.

**Repressor:** A protein that binds to a specific DNA site, decreasing the level of transcription of a gene. Repressors are capable of decreasing gene expression whether thay are upstream or downstream of the promoter.

**Restriction enzymes–restriction endonucleases:** Bacterial enzymes that recognize specific sequences in DNA, cutting the DNA only at those sites.

**Restriction fragment length polymorphisms (RFLPs):** Inherited differences in the sites at which restriction enzymes cut DNA, resulting in DNA fragments of different length.

**Restriction fragments:** Pieces of DNA that have been produced by exposure of a large piece of DNA to bacterial restriction endonucleases.

**Restriction map:** A diagram of DNA that defines DNA by its restriction enzyme sites.

**Restriction site:** That sequence of DNA that is cut by a specific restriction enzyme.

**Retrovirus:** An RNA virus that can reverse transcribe its RNA into DNA.

**RNA polymerase:** The enzyme that binds to the transcription complex assembled at the promoter and is responsible for copying, in a 5′ to 3′ direction, the antisense strand of DNA. Polymerases I and III catalyze production of rRNA and tRNA, respectively, whereas polymerase II produces an exact copy of the sense strand of DNA (hnRNA), which when processed to remove introns becomes mRNA.

**RNA:**

> **mRNA or messenger RNA:** The RNA that carries the genetic code from DNA to the ribosome for translation into proteins.
>
> **rRNA or ribosomal RNA:** the cytoplasmic RNA type on which the components of the protein synthetic machinery assemble. rRNA moves along mRNA, providing a positioning mechanism for tRNA to bring amino acids to the growing peptide chain.
>
> **tRNA or transfer RNA.** The RNA that carries specific amino acids to the ribosome for assembly of the polypeptide chain.

**Sense (strands):** The strand of DNA that contains the exact sequence as mRNA (except for the substitution of thymidine in DNA for uridine in RNA). This is the coding strand. The opposite strand is the noncoding antisense strand.

**Shuttle vector:** A vector that allows one to transfect DNA from one species of bacteria to another, for example, from mycobacteria to bacteria.

**Single-stranded conformational polymorphism (SSCP):** A method of determining variation in DNA sequence by separating DNA strands in a nondenaturing gel. Fragments with different secondary structures, introduced through mutations, assume different structure and migrate at different rates in the gel.

**Site-directed mutagenesis:** Altering one or more nucleotides at a specific place in the sequence of an oligonucleotide, in RNA or DNA.

**snRNPs:** Small nuclear ribonucleoproteins involved in splicing primary RNA transcripts.

**Southern blots:** DNA fragments separated by electrophoresis in a gel and transferred (blotted) to some sort of filter for subsequent hybridization with a labeled oligonucleotide probe.

**Splicesomes:** RNA-protein complexes in which RNA is processed by removal of introns and other information not required in mRNA for translation of proteins.

**Stable transfection:** Long-term, continuous expression of foreign DNA that has been introduced into a cell. It usually involves antibiotic selection and passage of those cells expressing the foreign gene that has been introduced.

**Start codon:** The nucleotide sequence AUG that signals for the addition of methionine to the ribosome and the beginning of translation, the start of protein formation.

**Sticky ends:** Overhang left between two DNA chains after exposure to a restriction enzyme. Some enzymes cut, leaving sticky ends that provide a site for tight ligation of or hybridization with complementary DNA sequences.

**Stop codon:** A sequence of three nucleotides that does not code for a specific amino acid (UAA, UGA, UAG) and thus signals that no additional amino acids will attach to the peptide being formed on the ribosome.

**Stringent:** Describes the conditions during hybridization of complementary strands of DNA or RNA. High stringency allows hybridization only when each nucleotide is complementary. Low stringency (low temperature or low salt concentration) allows hybridization when some nucleotides are not complementary.


**Tandem repeat:** DNA sequences that occur in multiple copies immediately adjacent to one another.

**Taq polymerase:** Polymerase used in PCR that is stable under extreme temperature changes and was originally derived from a thermal organism.

**Telomere:** Structures at the tip of a chromosome.

**Telophase:** The last stage of mitosis in which daughter chromosomes lie at opposite ends of the cell and a new nuclear envelope begins to form.

***trans*-Acting factors:** The proteins that bind to DNA at promoter, enhancer, or repressor sites to regulate transcription of DNA.

**Transcription:** The process of copying DNA into RNA. Everything that happens after DNA is copied is post-transcriptional.

**Transcription factors:** Proteins that affect the level of mRNA produced from DNA by either binding to DNA (*trans*-acting factors) or to other proteins.

**Transfection:** Introduction of foreign DNA into the nucleus of a cell, with the intent of expressing that DNA in the cell.

**Transformation:** The conversion of a normal cell to one with unregulated cell growth. Assessed by the ability of a cell to grow in soft agar, to form tumors in nude mice, and to continue growth after reaching the confluent state.

**Transgenes:** New genes that have been introduced into a host.

**Transgenic:** Animals created by introduction of foreign genes into the germ line.

**Transient transfection:** Short-term expression of foreign DNA in a cell versus stable transfection.

**Translation:** The process of making a protein from the nucleotide code in mRNA. The processing of the protein after it is made (translated) is post-translational.

**Translocation:** The exchange of genetic information between nonhomologous chromosomes.

**Transposon:** DNA elements that are capable of inserting themselves at various locations in the genome; also called mobile element.

**Triplet code:** The sequence of three nucleotides that signifies or codes for a specific amino acid.

**Uninformative mating or marker:** A mating or marker that cannot be used to establish linkage. For example, a microsatellite marker that is not polymorphic or different between parents.

**Untranslated regions of mRNA—5′ UT and 3′ UT:** The part of mRNA lying outside the open reading frame; therefore, it does not code for amino acids of the protein being made. The 5′ UT is the part of mRNA that lies between the beginning of mRNA and the methionine that signals the beginning of the open reading frame (start of protein formation). The 3′ UT lies between the stop site of translation and the poly A tail of mRNA.

**Upstream:** Sequences proceeding in a direction that is opposite the direction of expression—in DNA, sequences that lie 5′ from the site in question. Downstream of 3′ sequences lie in the opposite direction.

**Variable expression:** A trait in which a specific genotype will result in different phenotypes.

**Vector:** Anything used to transfer genetic material into a cell or tissue organism.

**Virion:** A viral particle.

**Western blot:** Protein fragments separated by electrophoresis in a gel and transferred (blotted) to some sort of filter for subsequent binding with a labeled antibody to that protein.

**X-linked:** Referring to genes carried on the X (female) chromosome, versus Y-linked.

**YAC vectors:** Yeast artificial chromosomes designed to carry up to 100 kb of DNA.

**Zoo blot:** A Southern or Northern blot using DNA or RNA from different species.

# Index

• • • • • • • • • • • • • • • • • • • • • • •

Page numbers in *italics* refer to illustrations;
numbers followed by t indicate tables.